中国本科医学教育标准
—临床医学专业

(2016 版)

教育部临床医学专业认证工作委员会

北京大学医学出版社

ZHONGGUO BENKE YIXUE JIAOYU BIAOZHUN:
LINCHUANGYIXUE ZHUANYE（2016）

图书在版编目（CIP）数据

中国本科医学教育标准——临床医学专业：2016版/教育部临床医学专业认证工作委员会编．—北京：北京大学医学出版社，2017.11（2022.7重印）

ISBN 978-7-5659-1701-1

Ⅰ．①中… Ⅱ．①教… Ⅲ．①临床医学–本科–医学教育–标准–中国　Ⅳ．①R-4

中国版本图书馆CIP数据核字（2017）第262583号

中国本科医学教育标准——临床医学专业（2016版）

主　　编：	教育部临床医学专业认证工作委员会
出版发行：	北京大学医学出版社
地　　址：	（100191）北京市海淀区学院路38号　北京大学医学部院内
电　　话：	发行部 010-82802230；图书邮购 010-82802495
网　　址：	http://www.pumpress.com.cn
E-mail：	booksale@bjmu.edu.cn
印　　刷：	中煤（北京）印务有限公司
经　　销：	新华书店
责任编辑：韩忠刚　　责任校对：金彤文　　责任印制：李　啸
开　　本：880 mm×1230 mm　1/32　印张：4.875　字数：68千字
版　　次：2017年11月第1版　2022年7月第5次印刷
书　　号：ISBN 978-7-5659-1701-1
定　　价：15.00元

版权所有，违者必究

（凡属质量问题请与本社发行部联系退换）

前　言

医学教育承载着培养医学卫生人才的使命，与全民健康息息相关。自2008年教育部和原卫生部颁布《本科医学教育标准—临床医学专业（试行）》以来，我国的本科临床医学教育认证工作逐步开展，成立了教育部医学教育认证专家委员会和教育部临床医学专业认证工作委员会，颁布了《临床医学专业认证指南（试行）》，初步建立了中国临床医学专业认证制度。在临床医学专业认证工作委员会与国际权威医学教育认证机构广泛交流与合作中，中国临床医学专业认证工作得到国际同行的关注与支持。

根据2012年《教育部卫生部关于实施临床医学教育综合改革的若干意见》（教高[2012]6号），我国将在2020年前"建立起具有中国特色与国际医学教育实质等效的医学专业认证制度"。为实现这一目标，教育部医学教育教学改革发展研究基地于2014年成立了"中国临床医学专业认证实施战略研究"课题组（以下简称课题组）。课题组根据国际医学教育发展趋势，并结合十年来积累的认证经验,对中国《本科医学教育标准—临床医学专业（试行）（2008版）》进行全面修订。此次标准的修订,主要依据世界医学教育联合会(World Federation for Medical Education, WFME)2012年修订的《本科医学教育质量改进全球标准》(*Basic Medical Education*:*WFME Global Standards for Quality Improvement*, The 2012 Revision),保留了中国《本科医学教育标准—临床医学专业(试行)(2008版)》中适用的内容,并确保中国标准与全球标准等效一致。此外还参照了澳大利亚医学理事会(Australian Medical Council, AMC)《本科临床医学专业评估与认证标准(2012版)》(*Standards for Assessment and Accreditation of Primary Medical Programs by the Australian Medical Council 2012*)、英国医学总会(General Medical Council, GMC)2009版《明日医生》(*Tomorrow's Doctors*)和美国医学教育联络委员会(The Liaison Committee on Medical Education, LCME)2013版《医学院校的职能与结构—临床医学专业认证标准》(*Functions and Structure of A Medical School*)等资料。课题组经过广泛的调研、专家咨询,历时两年,完成了《中国本科医学教育标准—临床医学专业(2016版)》的修订工作。

与2008版标准相比,本版标准分为基本标准(Basic Standards)和发展标准(Quality Development

Standards）。基本标准为所有举办临床医学专业本科教育的院校都必须达到的标准，用"必须"来表达。发展标准为国际所倡导的本科临床医学教育高标准，体现了医学教育发展的方向，用"应当"来表达，达成情况因各医学院校的不同发展阶段、资源状况和教育政策不同而有所不同。2016版标准的主领域仍为10个，亚领域由原来的44个调整为40个。条目包括113条基本标准和80条发展标准。为增加可读性，新标准采用了数字索引方式，同时为便于理解和操作，注释内容增加至92条。

本标准适用于临床医学专业本科教育阶段，是教育部临床医学专业认证的依据。本科医学教育是医学教育连续体中的第一阶段，其根本任务是为卫生保健机构培养完成医学基本训练，具有初步临床能力、终身学习能力和良好职业素质的医学毕业生。本科医学教育为学生毕业后继续深造和在各类卫生保健机构执业奠定必要的基础。医学毕业生胜任临床工作的专业能力需要在毕业后医学教育、继续职业发展和持续医疗实践中逐渐形成与提高。

本标准反映医学教育的国际趋势、国内现状和社会期待，是制订教育计划和规范教学管理的依据，各医学院校应参照此标准确立自身的办学定位，制订专业教育目标和教育计划，建立教育评价体系和质量保障机制。

本标准承认不同地区和学校之间的差异，尊重学校办学自主权。因此，它不作为评比排序的依据。在遵循医学教育基本规律的前提下，除必要的要求外，不对教学计划提出过多具体的、强制性的规定，为各校的发展及办学留下充分的空间。

应该着重强调的是，本标准以社会主义核心价值观（富强、民主、文明、和谐、自由、平等、公正、法治、爱国、敬业、诚信、友善）为基本准则，指导中国临床医学教育办学的全过程。

目　录

临床医学专业本科毕业生应达到的基本要求 ············ 1
　1．科学和学术领域 ················· 1
　2．临床能力领域 ·················· 2
　3．健康与社会领域 ················· 4
　4．职业素养领域 ·················· 5

临床医学专业本科医学教育办学标准 ············ 6
　1．宗旨与结果 ··················· 6
　2．教育计划 ···················· 13
　3．学业成绩考核 ·················· 25
　4．学生 ······················ 28
　5．教师 ······················ 32
　6．教育资源 ···················· 36
　7．教育评价 ···················· 44
　8．科学研究 ···················· 48
　9．管理与行政 ··················· 50
　10．持续改进 ···················· 54

临床医学专业本科毕业生应达到的基本要求

中国临床医学专业本科毕业生应树立正确的世界观、人生观、价值观，热爱祖国，忠于人民，遵纪守法，愿为祖国卫生事业的发展和人类身心健康奋斗终生。

中国临床医学专业本科毕业生应达到的基本要求分为四个领域：科学和学术、临床能力、健康与社会、职业素养。每所院校可根据自己的情况，对毕业生的预期结果提出更具体的要求。

医学教育是一个包括在校教育、毕业后教育和继续职业发展的连续过程。本科毕业生具备了一定的从业基础，为毕业后进一步发展做好充分的准备。但是医学生毕业时尚不具备丰富的临床经验，这就要求他们在日新月异的医学进步环境中保持其医学业务水平的持续更新，毕业生在校期间获得的教育培训以及掌握的科学方法将为他们终身学习与发展提供支撑。

1. 科学和学术领域

1.1 具备自然科学、人文社会科学、医学等学科的基础知识和掌握科学方法，并能用于指导未来的学习和医学实践。

1.2 能够应用医学等科学知识处理个体、群体和卫生系统中的问题。

1.3 能够描述生命各阶段疾病的病因、发病机制、自然病程、临床表现、诊断、治疗以及预后。

1.4 能够获取、甄别、理解并应用医学等科学文献中的证据。

1.5 能够掌握中国传统医学的基本特点和诊疗基本原则。

1.6 能够应用常用的科学方法，提出相应的科学问题并进行探讨。

2. 临床能力领域

2.1 具有良好的交流沟通能力，能够与患者及其家属、同行和其他卫生专业人员等进行有效的交流。

2.2 能够全面、系统、正确地采集病史。

2.3 能够系统、规范地进行体格检查及精神状态评价，规范地书写病历。

2.4 能够依据病史和体格检查中的发现，形成初步判断，并进行鉴别诊断，提出合理的治疗原则。

2.5 能够根据患者的病情、安全和成本效益等因素，选择适宜的临床检查方法并能说明其合理性，对检查结果能做出判断和解释。

2.6　能够选择并安全地实施各种常见的临床基本操作。

2.7　能够根据不断获取的证据做出临床判断和决策，在上级医生指导下确定进一步的诊疗方案并说明其合理性。

2.8　能够了解患者的问题、意见、关注点和偏好，使患者及其家属充分理解病情；努力同患者及其家属共同制订诊疗计划，并就诊疗方案的风险和益处进行沟通，促进良好的医患关系。

2.9　能够及时向患者及其家属/监护人提供相关信息，使他们在充分知情的前提下选择诊疗方案。

2.10　能够将疾病预防、早期发现、卫生保健和慢性疾病管理等知识和理念结合到临床实践中。

2.11　能够依据客观证据，提出安全、有效、经济的治疗方案。

2.12　能够发现并评价病情程度及变化，对需要紧急处理的患者进行急救处理。

2.13　能够掌握临终患者的治疗原则，沟通患者家属或监护人，避免不必要的检查或治疗。用对症、心理支持等姑息治疗的方法来达到人道主义的目的，提高舒适度并使患者获得应有的尊严。

2.14 能够在临床数据系统中有效地检索、解读和记录信息。

3. 健康与社会领域

3.1 具有保护并促进个体和人群健康的责任意识。

3.2 能够了解影响人群健康、疾病和有效治疗的因素，包括健康不公平和不平等的相关问题，文化、精神和社会价值观的多样化，以及社会经济、心理状态和自然环境因素。

3.3 能够以不同的角色进行有效沟通，如开展健康教育等。

3.4 解释和评估人群的健康检查和预防措施，包括人群健康状况的监测、患者随访、用药、康复治疗及其他方面的指导等。

3.5 能够了解医院医疗质量保障和医疗安全管理体系，明确自己的业务能力与权限，重视患者安全，及时识别对患者不利的危险因素。

3.6 能够了解我国医疗卫生系统的结构和功能，以及各组成部门的职能和相互关系，理解合理分配有限资源的原则，以满足个人、群体和国家的健康需求。

3.7 能够理解全球健康问题以及健康和疾病的决定因素。

4. 职业素养领域

4.1 能够根据《中国医师道德准则》为所有患者提供人道主义的医疗服务。

4.2 能够了解医疗卫生领域职业精神的内涵，在工作中养成同理心、尊重患者和提供优质服务等行为，树立真诚、正直、团队合作和领导力等素养。

4.3 能够掌握医学伦理学的主要原理，并将其应用于医疗服务中。能够与患者及其家属、同行和其他卫生专业人员等有效地沟通伦理问题。

4.4 能够了解影响医生健康的因素，如疲劳、压力和交叉感染等，并注意在医疗服务中有意识地控制这些因素，同时知晓自身健康对患者可能构成的风险。

4.5 能够了解并遵守医疗行业的基本法律法规和职业道德。

4.6 能够意识到自己专业知识的局限性，尊重其他卫生从业人员，并注重相互合作和学习。

4.7 树立自主学习、终身学习的观念，认识到持续自我完善的重要性，不断追求卓越。

临床医学专业本科医学教育办学标准

1. 宗旨与结果

1.1 宗旨

基本标准：

医学院校必须：

- 具有明确的办学宗旨，并让全校师生员工、医疗卫生机构等利益相关方知晓。(B* 1.1.1)
- 在宗旨中阐述医学生培养的目标及策略，使医学生在毕业时达到临床医学专业本科毕业生的基本要求。(B 1.1.2)
- 确保宗旨在相关法律框架内满足医疗服务体系和公众健康的需求，同时兼顾其他方面的社会责任。(B 1.1.3)

发展标准：

医学院校应当：

- 在宗旨中包括：

---

*注：
B 表示基本标准（Basic Standards），下同

- 医学研究目标。(Q^* 1.1.1)
- 全球卫生观念。(Q 1.1.2)

【注释】

- *宗旨*阐述医学院校及临床医学专业的总体框架，包括办学定位、办学理念、人才培养目标等。宗旨的制定应与学校的资源、管理相适应，同时考虑地方与国家、区域与全球对医学的期望和发展的需要，并体现学校历史文化积淀和发展愿景。办学定位应体现学校的办学类型、办学层次、服务面向、发展目标等；办学理念应体现学校人才培养的教育思想和观念。

- *医学院校*是指提供本科临床医学教育的教育机构，可独立建制，也可是综合性大学的一部分。医学院校还应包括附属医院及其他临床教学基地。医学院校不仅提供本科医学教育、开展研究、提供医疗服务，还可为医学教育的其他阶段或其他卫生相关行业提供教育方案和实施保障。

- *医疗卫生机构*包括公立、非公立医疗卫生服

---

*注：
Q 表示发展标准（Quality Development Standards），下同

务机构和医学研究机构。
- *满足公众健康的需求*是指与当地卫生及其相关部门进行沟通，通过调整课程计划来表明对当地公众健康问题的了解和关注。
- *社会责任*是指有意愿和能力通过提高医疗服务、医学教育及医学研究能力来满足社会、患者、卫生及其相关部门的需要，促进国家和国际医学事业的发展。社会责任应以尊重医学院校办学自主权为基础。超出医学院校权限的问题，尤其是健康卫生相关问题，医学院校可以通过表明态度、分析因果关系以及提出相应建议等方式展现其社会责任。
- *医学研究*包含生物医学、临床、行为和社会科学领域的所有与医学相关的科学研究。
- *全球卫生观念*是指对世界范围内主要健康问题的认知，包括对因种族差异、地域差别、贫富不均等所引起的不平等与不公平的健康问题的认识，以及为应对这些健康问题的挑战而需要开展的跨学科、跨部门、多行为体参与的全球卫生治理的认识。

1.2 宗旨制定过程的参与

基本标准：

医学院校必须：

- 保证学校校内主要利益相关方参与宗旨的形成。（B 1.2.1）

发展标准：

医学院校应当：

- 具有确保宗旨的制定有校外其他利益相关方参与的机制。（Q 1.2.1）

【注释】

- *校内主要利益相关方包括教师、学生、校/院领导和行政管理人员。*
- *校外其他利益相关方包括相关政府机构和主管部门、用人单位、社区和公众代表、学术和管理部门、专业学术团体、医学科研组织和毕业后教育机构的代表等。*

1.3 院校自主权和学术自由

基本标准：

医学院校必须：

- 拥有在符合相关法律、法规的前提下，制定和实施各项政策的自主权，尤其是在以下方面：
    - 课程计划的制定。（B 1.3.1）

- 课程计划实施所需资源的配置与使用。（B 1.3.2）
- 得到大学自然科学、人文社会科学等学科的学术支持。（B 1.3.3）

发展标准：

医学院校应当：

- 保证教师和学生有如下学术自由：
  - 在教学过程中从不同角度阐述和分析医学相关问题。（Q 1.3.1）
  - 在教学过程中选择适宜的教学资源。（Q 1.3.2）
  - 使用新的研究成果来说明具体问题。（Q 1.3.3）
- 加强大学人文社会学科及自然学科与医学学科间的融合。（Q 1.3.4）

【注释】

- *院校自主权*是指医学院校相对独立于政府或其他相关部门（区域及地方行政部门、私人合作方、行业协会、联盟和与临床医学专业相关的其他利益相关组织等），对招生、课程计划、评价考核、教师聘任及待遇、科研和资源配置等关键问题可以自主决策。院校自主权应以遵循法律法规和医学教育基本发展规律为前提。
- *学术自由*包括在法律允许下的教师和学生享有言论、学术探究及出版方面的自由。

1.4 教育结果

基本标准：

医学院校必须：

- 明确规定医学生毕业时在如下方面应达到的预期教育结果或表现：
  - 科学和学术、临床能力、健康与社会、职业素养四大领域的基本要求。（B 1.4.1）
  - 在医疗服务领域从业的必要基础。（B 1.4.2）
  - 在医疗服务领域的未来角色定位。（B 1.4.3）
  - 与后续住院医师规范化培训相关的要求。（B 1.4.4）
  - 终身学习的意愿和能力。（B 1.4.5）
  - 与社区健康、医疗服务领域需求和社会责任相关的其他要求。（B 1.4.6）
- 阐明学生在与同伴、教师、医疗服务领域其他从业者、患者及其家属相处时应有的恰当的行为方式。（B 1.4.7）

发展标准：

医学院校应当：

- 明确建立在校教育结果和毕业后教育之间的关系。（Q 1.4.1）
- 明确学生参与医学相关研究的要求以及期望的结果。（Q 1.4.2）
- 关注学生对于全球卫生状况认识的水平。（Q 1.4.3）

【注释】

- 教育结果是指对学生在各阶段学习结束后所应具备的科学和学术、临床能力、健康与社会、职业素养四方面的要求。包括掌握和理解以下相关知识：(1) 生物医学基础；(2) 包括公共卫生和健康教育与健康促进在内的预防医学；(3) 包括医学伦理学、卫生法学在内的行为和社会科学；(4) 临床医学，包括临床基本操作、沟通技能、疾病的诊断、治疗和预防、健康促进、康复、临床思维和解决问题等方面的临床能力；(5) 行医所需要的终身学习能力和胜任医生多重角色的职业素质。
- 学生恰当的行为方式应在行为准则、学生手册或相关文件中有具体要求。

- 终身学习是保持知识和技能不断更新的一种学习能力，可以通过评估和反思、参加继续医学教育（Continuing Medical Education，CME）或继续职业发展（Continuing Professional Development，CPD）等各类学习来实现。CME 专指针对医学实践知识和技能的继续教育，而 CPD 的概念更为宽泛，包括医生根据患者的需求，为保持、更新、发展或提高自身知识、技能和职业素质而从事的各种正式与非正式活动。
- 全球卫生是指超越国界范畴、需各国共同合作来解决的卫生相关问题。

2. 教育计划

2.1 课程计划与教学方法

基本标准：

医学院校必须：

- 依据医疗卫生服务的需要、医学科学的进步和医学模式的转变，制定与本校宗旨、目标、教育结果相适应的课程计划。（B 2.1.1）
- 课程计划体现加强基础、培养能力、注重素质和发展个性的原则。（B 2.1.2）

- 明确课程模式。(B 2.1.3)
- 阐明所采用的教学方法。(B 2.1.4)
- 培养学生自主学习和终身学习的能力。(B 2.1.5)
- 以平等的原则实施课程计划。(B 2.1.6)

发展标准:

医学院校应当:

- 确保课程计划和教学方法能够激发、培养和支持学生自主学习。(Q 2.1.1)

【注释】

- *课程计划*包括培养目标、预期结果、课程模式、课程设置(课程结构、组成、学分和时间分配)和考核方法等。
- *课程模式*可以以学科、器官系统、临床问题、案例等为基础。
- *教学方法*含教与学两个方面,包括课堂讲授、小组讨论、基于问题或案例的学习、同伴学习、实验、见(实)习、床旁教学、临床示教、临床技能训练以及社区实践和网络教学等。
- *平等的原则*是指所有提供教学和实践的人,都必须遵守公平性和多样化的原则,在保持教育和标准的稳定性时，院校教学管理、学生评价、培训的规章制度要充分考虑到学生的性别、民族、宗教、性取向、文化、社会背景等。
- 课程计划和教学方法需要以现代学习理论为基础。

2.2　科学方法教育

基本标准：

医学院校必须：

- 在整个课程计划中体现：
    - 科学方法原理，强调分析性、批判性思维能力的培养。（B 2.2.1）
    - 医学研究方法的训练。（B 2.2.2）
    - 循证医学思想的建立。（B 2.2.3）

发展标准：

医学院校应当：

- 鼓励学生参与科学研究，并将学生科研训练纳入课程计划。（Q 2.2.1）
- 将原创的或前沿的研究纳入教学过程中。（Q 2.2.2）
- 将科学方法原理、医学研究方法包括循证医学观念的教育贯穿整个人才培养过程。（Q 2.2.3）

2.3 人文社会科学和自然科学课程

基本标准：

医学院校必须：

- 在整个课程计划中覆盖下列领域的内容：
  - 人文社会科学，特别强调思想道德修养、医学伦理、卫生法学。（B 2.3.1）
  - 自然科学。（B 2.3.2）

发展标准：

医学院校应当：

- 将人文社会科学等融入医学专业教学中，重视职业素质的培养。调整并优化课程计划中人文社会科学的内容和权重，以适应：
  - 科学技术和临床医学发展。（Q 2.3.1）
  - 社会和医疗卫生体系当前和未来的需求。（Q 2.3.2）
  - 不断变化的人口和文化环境的需要。（Q 2.3.3）

【注释】

- 根据当地的需求、利益和传统，人文社会科学可以包括医学伦理学、卫生法学、医学心理学、医学社会学、卫生管理学等，每门课程涵盖的内容和深度取决于医学院校的教育目标。鼓励将人文社会科学知识内容有机地融入专业课程教学。
- *自然科学包括数学、物理、化学等。*

2.4　生物医学课程

基本标准：

医学院校必须：

- 在课程计划中开设生物医学基础课程，使学生全面了解医学科学知识，掌握基本概念和方法，并了解在临床中的应用。（B 2.4.1）

发展标准：

医学院校应当：

- 根据科学技术和医学发展以及社会对卫生保健服务的需求调整生物医学课程。（Q 2.4.1）

【注释】

- *生物医学课程包括人体解剖学、组织学与胚胎学、病理学、病原生物学、细胞生物学、医学遗传学、生物化学、生理学、医学免疫学、药理学、病理生理学等核心课程；以及分子生物学、神经生物学、生物物理、生物信息等拓展课程。以上课程也可以整合的形式呈现。核心课程应列为必修课程，拓展课程依培养目标的不同，可列为必修或选修*

课程。

2.5 公共卫生课程

基本标准：

医学院校必须：

- 安排公共卫生相关内容，培养学生的预防战略和公共卫生意识，使其掌握健康教育和健康促进的知识和技能。（B 2.5.1）

发展标准：

医学院校应当：

- 使学生了解全球卫生的状况，具有全球卫生意识。（Q 2.5.1）

【注释】

- 公共卫生相关内容包括医学统计学、流行病学、全球卫生、健康教育与健康促进、妇幼与儿少卫生学、社会医学、环境卫生、营养与食品卫生、劳动卫生与职业病学等。

2.6 临床医学课程

基本标准：

医学院校必须：

- 在课程计划中明确并涵盖临床学科内容，确保学生获得全面的临床知识、临床技能和职业能力，在毕业后能够承担相应的临床工作。

（B 2.6.1）
- 在临床环境中安排临床医学课程，确保学生有足够的时间接触患者，并做出合理的教学安排。（B 2.6.2）
- 保证理论授课和临床见习紧密结合。（B 2.6.3）
- 确保学生在与本校签有书面协议、具有教学资质的临床教学基地完成实习。（B 2.6.4）
- 保证毕业实习时间不少于48周，合理安排临床主要二级学科实习轮转即内科学、外科学、妇产科学、儿科学的实习时间。（B 2.6.5）
- 在临床实践中关注患者和学生的安全。（B 2.6.6）
- 课程计划包括与医生职责有关的交流技能的专门指导，包括与患者及其家属、同行及其他卫生行业人员的交流。（B 2.6.7）
- 安排适当的中国传统医学的基本思想和理论的相关课程。（B 2.6.8）
- 提倡早期接触临床。（B 2.6.9）

发展标准：

医学院校应当：
- 使每位学生都能够早期接触临床并更多地接

触患者。（Q 2.6.1）
- 根据不同学习阶段，合理安排学生进行不同内容的临床技能培训。（Q 2.6.2）
- 为医学生与其他专业的医疗人员及学生团队合作提供跨专业（Interprofessional Education，IPE）的学习机会。（Q 2.6.3）

【注释】

- *临床医学课程包括诊断学、内科学（含神经病学、传染病学等）、外科学（含外科学总论、麻醉学等）、妇产科学、儿科学、精神病学、眼科学、耳鼻咽喉与头颈外科学、皮肤性病学、口腔科学、中医学或其他民族医学、全科医学等核心课程；以及急诊医学、康复医学、老年医学、肿瘤学、舒缓医学、物理治疗、放射治疗学、临床药学（含抗生素合理使用）等拓展课程。临床医学课程也可以整合的形式呈现。核心课程与拓展课程的含义见 2.4 生物医学课程注释。*
- *临床技能包括病史采集、体格检查、沟通技能、辅助检查、诊断与鉴别诊断、制定和执行诊疗计划、临床基本操作等。*
- *职业能力包括患者处置能力、团队协作与交*

流能力、领导力、跨学科/专业合作能力等。
- *合理的教学安排*是指临床教学时间不少于整个课程计划时间的 1/2，在临床教学中实际接触患者的时间不少于整个课程计划时间的 1/3。
- *具有教学资质的临床教学基地*是指通过教育和/或卫生主管部门评估合格的临床教学基地。
- *临床主要二级学科实习轮转*包括内科（其中呼吸内科、心血管内科、消化内科应分别不少于 3 周）、外科（其中普通外科时间不应少于 6 周，且需同时包括胃肠外科和肝胆外科）、妇产科和儿科等科室轮转。
- *患者和学生的安全*指保证学生只承担他们能够胜任并符合相关规定的临床实践任务，并在过程中对学生进行监督管理，以保护患者的安全；同时保证学生安全的学习环境。
- *早期接触临床*指在基础医学学习阶段，有计划地在临床环境中安排临床相关内容的学习，主要包括医患沟通、病史采集、体格检查等。

2.7 课程计划的结构、组成

基本标准：

医学院校必须：

- 在课程计划中描述每门课程的内容、课程安

排的先后顺序以及其他课程要素，以保证生物医学课程、人文社会科学课程和临床科学课程之间的协调。（B 2.7.1）
- 课程设置应包括必修课程和选修课程，两者之间的比例可由学校根据实际情况确定。（B 2.7.2）

发展标准：

医学院校应当：
- 在课程计划中：
  - 进行相关学科课程的横向整合。（Q 2.7.1）
  - 进行临床医学与生物医学（基础医学）和人文社会科学的纵向整合。（Q 2.7.2）
  - 描述与替代医学的相互关系和作用。（Q 2.7.3）

【注释】
- *横向整合*指生物医学基础学科之间或临床学科之间的整合，如将生物医学基础学科的人体解剖学、生物化学和生理学进行整合；或将内科学与外科学进行整合，如消化内科学与胃肠外科学的整合、肾内科与泌尿外科学的整合。
- *纵向整合*指生物医学基础学科与临床学科的整合，如将新陈代谢紊乱和生物化学整合，或将心脏病学和心血管生理学整合。
- 替代医学是现代医学之外的医学理论与技术的总称。广义上包括中医、蒙医、藏医等，也包括诸如保健食品、食疗等非属传统医学的内容。

2.8 课程计划管理

基本标准：

医学院校必须：

- 设置教学（指导）委员会，在教学校/院长的领导下，负责审核和/或制定课程计划，以实现预期教育结果。（B 2.8.1）
- 在教学（指导）委员会中设有教师和学生代表。（B 2.8.2）

发展标准：

医学院校应当：

- 通过教学（指导）委员会制定课程改革方案并加以实施。（Q 2.8.1）
- 在教学（指导）委员会中设有其他利益相关方的代表。（Q 2.8.2）

【注释】

- 教学（指导）委员会在学校法规条例的允许范围内权衡各学科利益，宏观调控课程。教学（指导）委员会有权指导教学资源的配置，推进课程计划实施，评估学生和课程。
- *其他利益相关方*应该包括其他教学过程的参与者、实习医院和其他临床机构的代表、医学院校毕业生代表、社区及公众代表（如包括患者团体和组织在内的医疗服务体系的服务对象）或综合大学的其他学院。

2.9 与毕业后教育和继续医学教育的联系

基本标准：

医学院校必须：

- 确保课程计划与毕业后医学教育的有效衔接，并使毕业生具备接受继续医学教育的能力。（B 2.9.1）

发展标准：

医学院校应当：

- 根据毕业生质量调查结果和社会医疗服务需求等信息，及时修订、完善相应的课程计划。（Q 2.9.1）

【注释】

- *有效衔接*指根据医疗卫生问题，调整应达到的教育结果。有效衔接需要明确课程计划与毕业后各阶段医疗实践之间的关系；建立与卫生行政部门、用人单位、教师和学生的双向反馈机制。

3. 学业成绩考核

3.1 考核方法

基本标准：

医学院校必须：

- 围绕培养目标制定并公布学生学业成绩考核的总体原则和实施方案。内容包括考核的方式和频次、成绩构成、通过考核的分数、界定成绩等级的标准、允许重修次数等。（B 3.1.1）
- 确保考核覆盖科学和学术、临床实践能力、健康与社会、职业素养各个方面。（B 3.1.2）
- 根据不同的考核目的，采用广泛多样的考核方法和方式。（B 3.1.3）
- 建立并实施考核结果申诉制度。（B 3.1.4）

发展标准：

医学院校应当：

- 积极开展考核体系与方法的研究，探索新的、有效的考试方法并加以应用。（Q 3.1.1）
- 确保考核得到校外专家的指导与监督。（Q 3.1.2）

3.2 考核和学习之间的关系

基本标准：

医学院校必须：

- 明确采用的考核原则、方法与措施，能够达到以下要求：
  - 确保学生能够实现预期的教育结果。（B 3.2.1）
  - 有利于促进学生的学习。（B 3.2.2）
  - 做好终结性评价的同时，加强形成性评价的应用，并及时进行反馈，以便指导学生更好地学习。（B 3.2.3）

发展标准：

医学院校应当：

- 调整考核频次和类型，既鼓励基础知识的掌握又促进整合性学习。（Q 3.2.1）
- 基于考核结果，及时向学生提供具体的、有建设性的反馈意见。（Q 3.2.2）

【注释】

- 考核原则、方法与措施需对应培养目标整体设计，包括安排考试和其他测试的数量、时间，平衡笔试和口试的比例，根据规范和标准进行评判，鼓励使用客观结构化临床考试

(OSCE)、微型临床评估演练(Mini-CEX)、操作技能直接观察(DOPS)、计算机模拟病例考试(CCS)等。
- *终结性评价*是在教学活动结束后进行，用于判断教学目标是否达到预期结果的评价手段。终结性评价侧重于学生成绩和学习结果的评定。
- *形成性评价*强调教学过程与评价过程相结合，重视和强调教与学过程中的及时反馈和改进。形成性评价既有助于教师了解教学效果并优化教学，又有助于学生及时了解自己的学习状况并调整学习策略。
- 整合性学习可以通过实施综合性考核来促进，同时应确保对单个学科或单门课程领域的知识进行合理覆盖。

3.3 考试结果分析与反馈

基本标准：

医学院校必须：

- 在考试完成后进行基于教育测量学的考试分析。(B 3.3.1)
- 将考试分析结果及存在的问题以适当方式反馈给学生、教师和教学管理人员。(B 3.3.2)

发展标准：

医学院校应当：

- 将考试分析结果用于改进教与学。（Q 3.3.1）
- 加强考试的改革与研究（Q 3.3.2）

【注释】

- 考试分析包括试题难度和区分度、考试信度和效度，专业内容分析以及对考试整体结果的分析等。

4. 学生

4.1 招生政策及录取

基本标准：

医学院校必须：

- 根据国家的招生政策制定本校招生方案，并定期审核和调整。（B 4.1.1）
- 在保证招生质量的前提下，注意学生群体的多样性。（B 4.1.2）
- 在满足专业要求的前提下，不存在歧视和偏见。（B 4.1.3）
- 向社会公布招生章程，内容包括院校简介、专业设置、招生计划、收费标准、奖学金、申诉及监督机制等方面内容，明确说明学生

选拔过程并通过网络向考生公布课程计划。（B 4.1.4）
- 制定并实施学生转专业的制度。（B 4.1.5）

发展标准：

医学院校应当：
- 阐明学生录取原则与学校宗旨、课程计划及毕业生应达到的质量标准之间的关系。（Q 4.1.1）
- 具有明确的针对录取结果的申诉制度。（Q 4.1.2）

【注释】
- *招生方案应关注国家的相关政策，保证教育过程的同质性和公平性。*
- *学生选拔过程包括录取的基本原则和方法，如中学成绩、高考成绩、教育经历及学业状况、面试成绩、学习医学的动机、参加的社会实践活动、心理测试等。还应考虑到民族多样性、医疗实践多样性所导致的录取标准上的差异。*

4.2 招生规模

基本标准：

医学院校必须：
- 依据国家相关政策、社会医疗需求和学校的

教育资源合理确定招生规模。（B 4.2.1）

发展标准：

医学院校应当：

- 在审核和调整招生规模时，考虑利益相关方的意见。（Q 4.2.1）

【注释】

- *社会医疗需求包括国家和区域对医学人才的需要，也包括性别、民族和其他社会需求（人群的社会文化和语言特点），如为弱势学生及少数民族学生制定特殊招生和录取政策等。*
- *教育资源应考虑到医学相关专业学生对临床教育资源的占用。*
- *利益相关方包括教育和卫生行政部门人员、医疗卫生机构人员、教师、学生和公众代表等。*

4.3 学生咨询与支持

基本标准：

医学院校必须：

- 建立有效的学业咨询与支持体系。（B 4.3.1）
- 对学生学习、生活、勤工助学、就业等方面提供必需的支持服务。（B 4.3.2）
- 建立有效的心理咨询体系。（B 4.3.3）
- 配置学生支持服务所需的资源。（B 4.3.4）

- 确保学生接受咨询与支持的隐私权不受侵犯，不泄露学生的隐私。(B 4.3.5)

发展标准：

医学院校应当：

- 根据学生学业进展情况，提供个性化学业指导和咨询。(Q 4.3.1)
- 为学生提供职业指导和规划。(Q 4.3.2)

【注释】

- *学业咨询应包括课程的选择、住院医师阶段的准备以及就业指导等方面的内容。*
- *学生支持服务包括医疗服务、就业指导、为学生包括残障学生提供合理的住宿，执行奖学金、贷学金、助学金、困难补助等助学制度，为学生提供经济帮助。*
- *个性化学业指导和咨询除学习指导外，包括为每位学生或学生小组指定学术导师。*

4.4　学生代表

基本标准：

医学院校必须：

- 制定和实施有关政策，确保学生代表能够参与课程计划的设计、管理和考核以及其他与学生有关的事宜。(B 4.4.1)

- 支持学生依法成立学生社团组织，指导鼓励学生开展有益的社团活动，并为之提供必要的设备和场所、技术和资金支持。(B 4.4.2)

发展标准：

医学院校应当：

- 在学校的相关委员会、团体和相关社会机构中设立学生代表并发挥作用。(Q 4.4.1)

【注释】

- 学生社团组织包括学生自我管理、自我教育、自我服务的相关团体。

5. 教师

5.1 教师聘任与遴选政策

基本标准：

医学院校必须：

- 制定和实施教师资格认定制度和教师聘任制度，确保师资适应教学、科研、社会服务的需求。(B 5.1.1)
- 根据学校的目标定位和办学规模，配备数量足够、结构合理的具有教学资质的教师队伍。(B 5.1.2)
- 聘任教师时应设定其职责范围，并确保职责

范围内教学、科研和社会服务之间的比例与平衡。(B 5.1.3)
- 阐明教师在教学、科研和社会服务的业绩标准,定期对教师的业绩进行评价。(B 5.1.4)
- 有相应的机制保证教学业绩的评价结果在职称评定、职务晋升、岗位聘任等环节发挥作用。(B 5.1.5)

发展标准:

医学院校应当:
- 在制定教师的聘任政策时考虑学校办学宗旨、改革与发展的需求。(Q 5.1.1)
- 在制定教师的聘任政策时考虑人员经费和资源的合理有效利用,以利于教学、科研和社会服务均衡发展。(Q 5.1.2)

【注释】
- *教师聘任及遴选政策要确保足够数量和高质量的生物医学基础专业人员、行为与社会科学专业人员以及临床医生参与完成课程计划规定的授课任务。*
- *具有教学资质的教师指的是被聘任教师必须具有良好的职业道德及与其学术等级相称的学术水平和教学能力,能够承担相应的课程和规定*

的教学任务，并得到相关教育部门的认可。非医学教育背景教师对医学教育应有所了解。
- 业绩标准可以依据教师资质、专业经验、教学奖励、科研成果、学生评价、同行评价等方面衡量。

5.2 教师活动与教师发展政策

基本标准：

医学院校必须：

- 制定教师培训、晋升、支持和评价等政策并能有效实施，确保人才培养的中心地位。这些政策应当：
    - 保障教师的合法权利。（B 5.2.1）
    - 认可和支持教师的专业发展活动。（B 5.2.2）
    - 鼓励教师将临床经验和科研成果应用于教学。（B 5.2.3）
    - 保证教师直接参与课程计划和教育管理决策的制订。（B 5.2.4）
    - 保证教师对人才培养目标、课程计划有充分的了解。（B 5.2.5）
    - 努力促进教师的交流。（B 5.2.6）
    - 努力使教师具备并保持胜任教学工作的能力。（B 5.2.7）

- 保证教师的教学、科研和社会服务职能的平衡。（B 5.2.8）

发展标准：

医学院校应当：

- 重视课程和教学模式的差异性，根据课程的需求，配置合理的师资。（Q 5.2.1）
- 建立教师参与学校/院管理和政策制定的机制。（Q 5.2.2）

【注释】

- *教师活动与教师发展涉及全体教师，不仅包括新教师，也包括所有基础和临床的教师。*
- *教师发展应强调教师教学能力的提升，可由专门的教学支持和发展部门为教师提供教育理念、课程设计、教学方法、教学评价等方面的培训。*
- *教育管理决策应包括招生、学生事务等。除此之外，教师也应当参与学校其他重要任务的决策。*
- *教师对课程计划有充分的了解包括了解教学方法、全部课程内容、考核方式，从而促进学科间的合作和整合，对学生进行适当的学习指导。*

- *教师的交流应包括教师在本学科领域内、学科领域间的交流，重视医学院内临床医学与基础医学教师间的沟通交流。*
- *胜任教学工作的能力表现为能够适应学校的教育目标，遵守教学的基本原则，设计适当的教学活动和学生成绩评定方式。*
- *教学、科研和社会服务职能的平衡指教师合理安排相关工作的时间，社会服务职能包括卫生保健系统中的临床服务、学生指导、行政管理及其他社会服务工作。*

6. 教育资源

6.1 教育预算与资源配置

基本标准：

医学院校必须：

- 有可靠的经费筹措渠道，保证稳定的教育经费来源。（B 6.1.1）
- 教育经费与资源足以支持完成医学教育计划，实现学校的办学目标。（B 6.1.2）

发展标准：

医学院校应当：

- 能够多渠道筹措教育经费。（Q 6.1.1）

- 教育经费可以支持对医学教育改革和发展的探索。(Q 6.1.2)

【注释】
- 教育经费中学校收取的学费应当按照国家有关规定管理和使用,其中教学经费及其所占学校当年财务决算的比例必须达到国家有关规定的要求。鉴于医学教育高成本的特点,应增加医学生人均拨款,以满足教学要求。
- 多渠道筹措教育经费包括政府拨款、学费收入、社会团体和公民个人投入、捐赠和基金收入、附属/教学医院支持、校办产业和社会服务收入等多元化筹资方式。

6.2 基础设施

基本标准:

医学院校必须:

- 提供足够的基础设施,确保课程计划得以实施。(B 6.2.1)
- 提供安全的学习环境,保证师生和患者的安全。(B 6.2.2)
- 为学生提供进行临床模拟训练的场所和设备。(B 6.2.3)

发展标准：

医学院校应当：

- 定期更新、添加和拓展基础设施以改善学习环境，并使其与开展的教育项目相匹配。（Q 6.2.1）
- 更新并有效利用临床模拟设备，开展临床模拟情境教学。（Q 6.2.2）

【注释】

- 基础设施应包括各类教室及多媒体设备、小组讨论（学习）室、基础实验室（含实验设备、材料和标本）、临床技能中心及设备、临床示教室、图书馆、信息技术和网络资源等，并为学生提供住宿、饮食、文体活动等设施。
- 安全的学习环境应包括提供针对有害物质、标本和微生物的必要信息提示与保护措施、实验室安全条例及安全设备。并公布其处理突发事件和防灾状态的制度和程序。

6.3 临床教学资源

基本标准：

医学院校必须：

- 拥有直属的综合性三级甲等附属医院。（B 6.3.1）

- 确保足够的临床教学基地和资源，满足临床教学需要，医学类专业在校学生与病床总数比应小于1∶1。(B 6.3.2)
- 有足够的师资对学生的临床实践进行指导。(B 6.3.3)

发展标准：

医学院校应当：

- 持续评价、调整并更新临床教学资源，以满足教学与社会卫生服务需求。(Q 6.3.1)

【注释】

- *附属医院*是医学院的组成部分，与医学院校有隶属关系。
- *临床教学基地*除附属医院以外，还包括教学医院、实习医院和社区卫生实践基地。附属医院和大学有行政隶属关系，教学医院、实习医院等与大学无行政隶属关系。教学医院必须符合下列条件：有省级政府部门认可作为医学院校临床教学基地的资质；学校和医院双方有书面协议；有能力、有责任承担包括临床理论课、见习和实习在内的全程临床教学任务；有完善的临床教学规章制度、教学组织机构和教学团队等。

- *临床教学资源除临床教学设施和设备之外，还包括足够的患者和病种数量。*
- *医学类专业包括临床医学、口腔医学、麻醉学、医学影像学、眼视光医学、精神医学、放射医学、中医学、中西医临床医学、基础医学、法医学、预防医学等授予医学学士学位的专业。医学类专业在校学生包括上述专业的本科生、中／英文授课的留学生和专科生。*
- *病床总数指附属医院床位数与教学医院床位数之和，其中附属医院床位数是指参与临床专业教学的附属综合医院和附属专科医院的床位数之和。教学医院床位数是指承担全程临床教学并有一届临床医学专业毕业生的教学医院的床位数之和，但不包括承担部分教学的专科医院的床位数。医院的床位数为医院上一年向卫生部门呈报的年终统计报表床位数，如实际开放的床位数低于编制床位数，则按实际计算。*
- *评价临床教学资源包括从环境、设备、患者和病种数量、医疗卫生服务及其监督与管理等方面进行评价，衡量是否满足教学需求。*

还需要考虑附属医院或者教学医院承担外校医学类专业学生占用资源情况。

6.4 信息技术服务

基本标准：

医学院校必须：

- 拥有足够的信息技术基础设施和支持服务系统，方便学生使用。（B 6.4.1）
- 制定并实施相关政策，确保现代信息技术与资源能有效地服务于教学，保证课程计划的落实。（B 6.4.2）

发展标准：

医学院校应当：

- 保证师生能够有效利用现有的信息技术并探索新技术，以支持自主学习。（Q 6.4.1）
- 保证学生能够最大程度地获取患者的相关信息及使用医疗信息系统。（Q 6.4.2）

【注释】

- *有效利用现有的信息技术*是指通过现代信息技术手段构建校园数字化学习平台，使学生能够利用所有的教学资源，为学生利用信息技术提供支持。信息和通讯技术有助于学生循证医学和终身学习意识的培养，为学生接受未来的继续职业发展（CPD）或继续医学教育（CME）做好充分准备。

6.5 教育专家

基本标准：

医学院校必须：

- 有制度和措施保证教育专家参与医学教育重要问题的决策，包括课程计划的制订、教学方法和考核方式的选择与调整改革等。（B 6.5.1）

发展标准：

医学院校应当：

- 充分发挥教育专家在教师成长中的作用。（Q 6.5.1）
- 重视培养校内教育专家医学教育研究和评价的能力。（Q 6.5.2）

【注释】

- *教育专家*是指熟悉并研究医学教育问题、过程和实践并具有先进教育理念的人才，可以包括具有不同学科背景的教师、医生、管理者、研究人员等。教育专家可来自校内，也可以从其他高校或机构聘请。

6.6 教育交流

基本标准：

医学院校必须：

- 制定并实施与国内或国际其他教育机构合作的相关政策。(B 6.6.1)
- 提供适当资源，促进学生、教师和管理人员等进行地区间及国际间的交流。(B 6.6.2)

发展标准：

医学院校应当：

- 制定并实施课程学分转换的相关政策。(Q 6.6.1)
- 考虑教师及学生的需求，尊重各方的风俗习惯和文化背景等伦理原则，有目的地组织交流活动。(Q 6.6.2)

【注释】

- 课程学分转换需在学校之间签署双方互认协议，确保满足本校课程计划的要求。制定公开透明的学分体系、详细描述课程要求有利于推进课程学分转换和学生交流。

7. 教育评价

7.1 教育监督与评价机制

基本标准:

医学院校必须:

- 建立教育监督与评价的机制,强调对教育计划、过程及结果的监督与评价。(B 7.1.1)
- 依据专业的质量标准,对教育过程各环节提出具体的要求。(B 7.1.2)
- 将相关监督与评价结果用于课程计划的改进。(B 7.1.3)
- 使学校师生与管理人员了解教育监督与评价体系。(B 7.1.4)

发展标准:

医学院校应当:

- 定期对教育计划进行全面评估,包括实施教学的环境、课程计划的具体内容、总体结果和社会责任等。(Q 7.1.1)
- 对学生的学习进行跟踪评价,如学习过程、学习能力变化、生活和学术上的支持等,并及时反馈给学生。(Q 7.1.2)
- 培训相关评价人员,使其能够选择和使用合

适、有效的评价方法。(Q 7.1.3)

【注释】

- *教育评价指根据相应的标准，运用科学手段，通过系统的收集信息资料和分析整理，对教育计划、教育过程和教育结果进行的质量判断，为提高教育质量和教育决策提供依据的过程。信息资料可包括大学或医学院的质量评估文件，如政策条例、手册、会议纪要、与其他教育机构的联合协议、监督报告和学生评价结果等。*
- *教育监督指针对课程主要环节的日常资料收集，目的在于保证教育活动的正常运行，并及时发现需要干预的环节。*
- *实施教学的环境包括医学院校的组织架构和资源以及学习环境和文化氛围。*
- *课程计划的具体内容包括课程描述、教学与学习的方法、临床轮转和学生考核方法。*
- *总体结果通过如国家医师资格考试、住院医师规范化培训合格考试、职业选择、就业单位及毕业后表现等指标来衡量，可作为课程改进的基础。*

7.2 教师和学生反馈

基本标准：

医学院校必须：

- 采用多种评价方式，系统地搜集信息，分析教师和学生的反馈并做出回复。（B 7.2.1）

发展标准：

医学院校应当：

- 将反馈结果用于教育计划的改进并取得成效。（Q 7.2.1）

【注释】

- 反馈不仅包括教育过程、教育结果方面的信息，还应包括学校的政策措施、教师和学生的各种违纪行为的处理等。

7.3 学生表现

基本标准：

医学院校必须：

- 将学生在校期间和毕业后的表现与学校办学宗旨、预期教育结果、课程计划和提供的教育资源联系起来。（B 7.3.1）

发展标准：

医学院校应当：

- 将在校生和毕业生质量的分析结果作为制定

招生政策、课程计划修订、学生咨询服务的依据。(Q 7.3.1)

【注释】
- *毕业生质量的分析应围绕毕业生基本要求的内容进行*，包括毕业生的职业选择、临床实践的表现和晋升等信息的收集、整理和分析。

7.4 利益相关方的参与

基本标准：

医学院校必须：
- 有教师、学生和行政管理部门人员等校内利益相关方参与教育监督与评价。(B 7.4.1)

发展标准：

医学院校应当：
- 鼓励校外利益相关方参与对课程计划的监督与评价，了解评估的结果。(Q 7.4.1)
- 征询校外利益相关方对毕业生质量、课程计划的反馈意见。(Q 7.4.2)

【注释】
- *校外利益相关方*包括其他学术和管理人员代表、社区和公众代表（如医疗服务的对象）、教育和卫生行政部门以及医疗卫生机构和毕业后教育工作者等。

8. 科学研究

8.1 教学与科学研究

基本标准：

医学院校必须：

- 制定并实施相关政策，促进科研与教学协调发展。（B 8.1.1）
- 将科学研究和学术成果作为制定与实施教育计划的支撑。（B 8.1.2）
- 加强对医学教育及管理的研究，为教学改革与发展提供理论依据。（B 8.1.3）

发展标准：

医学院校应当：

- 将科研活动、科研成果引入教学过程，以培养学生的科学思维、科学方法及科学精神，保证科学研究和教学之间的良性互动。（Q 8.1.1）

【注释】

- 科学研究包括在生物医学、临床医学、行为与社会科学领域的科研活动。科学研究促进教学体现在教学中加强科研方法和循证医学的学习。

8.2 教师科研

基本标准：

医学院校必须：

- 为教师提供基本的科学研究条件，鼓励教师开展科学研究，促进科研与教学相结合。（B 8.2.1）
- 要求教师具备相应的科学研究能力。（B 8.2.2）

发展标准：

医学院校应当：

- 鼓励教师积极参与医学教育研究，提升教学能力。（Q 8.2.1）

8.3 学生科研

基本标准：

医学院校必须：

- 将科学研究活动作为培养学生科学素养和创新思维的重要途径，采取积极、有效措施为学生创造参与科学研究的机会与条件。（B 8.3.1）
- 在课程计划中安排综合性、设计性实验，开设学术讲座、组织科研小组等，开展有利于培养学生科研能力的活动。（B 8.3.2）

发展标准：

医学院校应当：

- 为学生提供科学研究经费，以满足学生参与科学研究的需要。（Q 8.3.1）

9. 管理与行政

9.1 管理

基本标准：

医学院校必须：

- 明确阐述管理结构，界定管理职能，建立大学、医学院及附属医院之间的有效管理机制，确保医教研的协调发展。（B 9.1.1）
- 设立相应委员会，审议课程计划、教学改革及科学研究等重要事项。委员会应该包括院校领导、师生代表和管理人员等校内利益相关方代表。（B 9.1.2）

发展标准：

医学院校应当：

- 在相应委员会中包含上级行政主管部门、医疗卫生机构及社会公众等校外利益相关方代表。（Q 9.1.1）

- 保证医学教育管理工作和决策过程的透明性。(Q 9.1.2)

【注释】

- *管理*主要涉及政策制定、决策过程及政策执行的监管。学校政策和教育教学政策通常涵盖医学院校办学宗旨、课程计划、招生政策、员工招聘与选拔等方面的规定以及与医疗卫生部门及其他校外机构的联系与合作方面的决策。
- *委员会*组成人员应有广泛的代表性。委员会的活动应明确组织者或召集人，相关人员参与活动的时间、内容应有记录。
- *透明性*可通过简讯、网络信息和会议报道等方式得以实现。

9.2 医学院校与教学管理部门领导

基本标准：

医学院校必须：

- 明确阐述医学院校领导对医学教育的管理职责和权限，并确保执行。(B 9.2.1)
- 保证教学管理部门领导任职时间相对稳定。(B 9.2.2)

- 重视医学教育主管领导的专业教育背景。（B 9.2.3）

发展标准：

医学院校应当：

- 定期评估医学院校领导在实现办学目标和预期教育结果等方面的业绩。（Q 9.2.1）

【注释】

- 医学院校领导指管理机构和行政机构内部，负责教学、科研和服务等方面学术事宜决策的人员，包括院长、副院长、教务处长等。
- 管理职责和权限特别强调医学院校教学主管领导在组织制订和实施课程计划、合理调配教育资源方面的权利。

9.3 行政人员及管理

基本标准：

医学院校必须：

- 建立结构合理、理念先进的行政管理队伍，确保课程计划及其他教学活动的顺利实施。（B 9.3.1）
- 建立科学的管理制度及操作程序，确保资源合理配置。（B 9.3.2）

发展标准：

医学院校应当：

- 建立内部管理质量保障机制，并定期审核。（Q 9.3.1）

【注释】

- *内部管理质量保障机制包括对管理工作的评估，以改进管理工作。*

9.4 与医疗卫生机构、行政管理部门的相互关系

基本标准：

医学院校必须：

- 与行政管理部门加强联系和交流，争取各方面对人才培养的支持。（B 9.4.1）
- 与相关医疗卫生机构签署协议，保证教学的顺利实施。（B 9.4.2）

发展标准：

医学院校应当：

- 与医疗卫生机构和行政管理部门开展更广泛的合作与交流，保证可持续发展。（Q 9.4.1）

【注释】

- *相关医疗卫生机构包含公立或私立医疗服务机构、医学研究机构、健康促进组织、疾病防控机构。*

- 广泛的合作与交流指达成正式协议，明确合作的内容与形式并开展合作项目等。

10. 持续改进

基本标准：

医学院校必须：

- 定期回顾和评估自身发展，明确自身存在的问题并持续改进。（B 10.0.1）

发展标准：

医学院校应当：

- 基于前瞻性研究、医学教育文献回顾、各类评估评价结果等不断反思，持续改进。（Q 10.0.1）
- 通过改革形成相应的政策和措施，并与既往经验、现状和未来发展相适应。（Q 10.0.2）
- 在持续发展中主要关注以下方面：
    - 调整医学院校的办学宗旨和预期教育结果，使之与科学、社会经济和文化发展相适应。（Q 10.0.3）
    - 根据毕业生工作岗位的需求调整预期教育结果，调整内容应包括临床技能、公共卫生培训和医疗实践等。（Q 10.0.4）

- 调整课程模式和教学方法，保证两者之间的合理性和相关性。（Q 10.0.5）
- 调整课程内容及各部分之间的关系，使之与生物医学、临床医学、行为和社会科学的发展以及人口特点、群体健康与疾病模式、社会经济和文化环境的改变相适应。通过调整，使相关知识、概念和方法得到更新。（Q 10.0.6）
- 根据预期教育结果以及教学方法的变化，确定学生考核的原则、方法及措施。（Q 10.0.7）
- 调整招生政策、选拔方法与录取规模，使之适应预期结果、人力资源需求和医学教育体系改变的需求。（Q 10.0.8）
- 根据改革和发展的需求，调整教师聘用和教师发展政策，更新教育资源，优化组织结构以及管理行政工作。（Q 10.0.9）
- 完善对教学过程的监督和评价，使评价结果及时展现教学目标的达成情况。（Q 10.0.10）

Standards for Basic Medical Education in China

(The 2016 Revision)

Working Committee for the Accreditation of Medical Education, Ministry of Education, P. R. China

Peking University Medical Press

Preface

Medical education programs in China carry out the mission of training competent health professionals, thusly closely related to the health outcomes of all citizens. Since the Ministry of Education (MOE) and the former Ministry of Health issued *Standards for Basic Medical Education (for Trial Implementation)* in 2008, the accreditation system of basic medical education in China has been gradually developed. The Expert Committee for the Accreditation of Medical Education and the Working Committee for the Accreditation of Medical Education (WCAME) of the MOE have been established, the official *Guidelines for Accreditation of Medical Education (for Trial Implementation)* has been released, and the accreditation activities have been steadily conducted. With the wide and in-depth interaction and cooperation between the WCAME and other international accreditation bodies of medical education, the accreditation of basic medical education in China has gained substantial attention and support from the international counterparts.

According to the "Opinions on the Implementation of Comprehensive Reforms of Medical Education by *the Ministry of Education and the Ministry of Health in 2012" (Jiao Gao [2012] No.6)*, China will "establish an accreditation system of medical education with Chinese characteristics and equivalent to the international practices" by 2020. In a bid to achieve this goal, the Research Institute for the Reform and Development of Medical Education of the MOE established the research team on "strategic study on the implementation of accreditation of basic medical education in China" (hereinafter referred to as research team) in 2014. In the light of the trend of international medical education and the accreditation experience acquired over the past decade, the research team carried out a comprehensive revision of the *Standards for Basic Medical Education (for Trial Implementation)* and finalized the *2016 Revision* through thorough investigation and consultations. This revision, retaining appropriate contents in the *Standards for Basic Medical Education (for Trial Implementation)*, was mainly based on the Basic Medical Education: *WFME Global Standards for Quality Improvement (the 2012 Revision)* issued by the World Federation for Medical Education (WFME) in 2012, with reference to the *Standards for Assessment and Accreditation of Primary Medical Programs by the Australian Medical Council 2012* by the Australian Medical Council (AMC), *Tomorrow's Doctors 2009* by the General Medical Council (GMC) and *Functions and Structure of A Medical School 2013* by the Liaison Committee on Medical Education (LCME).

In contrast to the original 2008 version, the 2016 revision incorporates standards at two levels of attainment, the basic standard and quality development standard. The basic *standard* in principle must be met by every medical school providing basic medical education, which is expressed with a "must" statement. The quality development *standard* is in accordance with international consensus on the best practices in basic medical education hereby representing the trend of development, which is expressed with a "should" statement. Fulfillment of quality development standards will vary with the phases of development, available resources, educational policy and other conditions of the medical schools. The set of standards in the 2016 revision is grouped into 10 areas as the original 2008 version, but with a total of 40 instead of 44 sub-areas. There are a total of 113 basic and 80 quality development standards in the 2016 revision. To enhance the readability, the 2016 revision adopts a digital index. And the number of annotations also increases to 92, to facilitate easier comprehension and implementation of reform measures.

The 2016 revision, applicable to basic medical education in China, serves as the basis for its accreditation. As the first stage of the continuum of medical education, basic medical education is to develop a medical graduate with foundational clinical ability, life-long learning capability and desired quality of professionalism through complete medical training processes. It lays an essential foundation for further learning and practice in various health care institutions for the medical students. The professional capability of medical graduates in clinical practices needs to be gradually formed and improved in the postgraduate medical education, the continuing professional development and the continuing medical practices.

The 2016 revision reflects the international trend,

taking the consideration of the domestic needs and societal expectations of medical education systems in China, which is the basis for formulating curricular programs and standardizing educational management. Each medical school is required to determine its educational objectives, formulate its expected educational outcomes and curriculum, and establish its quality assurance system based on its own characteristics and standards in the 2016 revision.

The revision also acknowledges the differences in geographic locations and among institutions, and respects the autonomy of each medical school. Therefore, it cannot be used for the ranking of medical schools. With the prerequisite of adhering to the basic principles of medical education, the revision does not set many specific and compulsory requirements apart from essential ones, so that there is sufficient space for the development and operations of each institution.

It should be highlighted that the revision upholds the core values of socialism (prosperity, democracy, civility, harmony, freedom, equality, justice, the rule of law, patriotism, dedication, integrity and friendship) as the basic principle to guide the entire course of medical education in China.

Contents

Graduate Outcomes of Basic Medical Education ··· **67**
  1. Science and Scholarship: the medical graduate as a scientist and a scholar ·················· 68
  2. Clinical Practice: the medical graduate as a practitioner ································· 69
  3. Health and Society: the medical graduate as a health advocate ····························· 71
  4. Professionalism: the medical graduate as a professional ································· 73

Standards for Basic Medical Education in China ··· **75**
  1. Mission and Outcomes ················· 75
  2. Education Programme ················· 85
  3. Assessment of Students ················ 101
  4. Students ··························· 106
  5. Academic Staff/Faculty ················ 112
  6. Educational Resources ················ 118
  7. Programme Evaluation ················ 128

8. Scientific Research ································ 134
9. Governance and Administration ················· 137
10. Continuous Development ······················· 142

Graduate Outcomes of Basic Medical Education

The graduates of basic medical education in China should develop the correct views of the world, life and values. They should possess core values of patriotism and collectivism, and be loyal to the people. Besides abiding by the law, they should be willing to make a lifetime dedication to the development of the health care service of the country and the physical and mental well-being of mankind.

The graduate outcomes of basic medical education in China are presented in four domains: Science and Scholarship, Clinical Practice, Health and Society, and Professionalism. More specific requirements of the expected outcomes should be formulated by each institution on the basis of its own characteristics.

Medical education is a continuum covering basic education, postgraduate education and continuing professional development. At the end of basic medical education, the graduates will possess essential foundations for medical practice and be fully prepared for their further learning and development after graduation. However, the graduates do not have rich clinical experiences upon graduation, which requires them to keep upgrading their professional competence in time with the advancing pace in medicine. This requires the graduates to be mastering the scientific approaches and acquiring the ability for lifelong learning during their study in the medical school.

1. Science and Scholarship: the medical graduate as a scientist and a scholar

At the end of basic medical education, graduates are able to:

1.1 Possess the fundamental knowledge of the disciplines such as natural sciences, humanities and social sciences and medicine, and apply scientific methods, which will be applicable in future study and medical practices.

1.2 Apply medical and scientific knowledge to individual patients, populations and the health systems.

1.3 Describe the etiology, pathology, natural history, clinical features, diagnosis, treatment and prognosis of common presentations at all stages of life.

1.4 Access, critically appraise, interpret and apply evidence from the medical and scientific literature.

1.5 Master the basic features of traditional Chinese medicine and its basic principle of diagnosis and treatment.

1.6 Apply knowledge of common scientific methods to formulate relevant research questions.

2. Clinical Practice: the medical graduate as a practitioner

At the end of basic medical education, graduates are able to:

2.1 Conduct effective communications with patients, their family members, colleagues and health professionals of other disciplines.

2.2 Take a medical history in a proper, comprehensive and systematic way.

2.3 Perform a full and accurate physical examination, including a mental state examination, and write medical records as required.

2.4 Integrate and interpret findings from the medical history and examination, to arrive at an initial assessment including a relevant differential diagnosis. Discriminate between possible differential diagnoses and propose rational management principles.

2.5 Select and justify common investigations, with regard to the pathological basis of disease, utility, safety and cost effectiveness, and interpret the results.

2.6 Select and perform a range of common procedures safely.

2.7 Make clinical judgements and decisions based on available evidence. Identify and justify relevant management options under the guidance of supervising physicians.

2.8 Understand patients' questions, views, concerns and preferences, and ensure patients' full understanding of their situations and options. Involve patients in the decision-making and planning of their treatments, including communicating risks and benefits of management options.

2.9 Provide information to patients, and family carers where relevant, to enable them to make fully informed choices among various diagnostic, therapeutic and management options.

2.10 Integrate prevention, early detection, health

maintenance and chronic disease management where relevant into clinical practices.

2.11 Prescribe medications safely, effectively and economically based on objective evidence.

2.12 Recognise and assess deteriorating and critically unwell patients who require immediate care. Perform common emergency and life support procedures.

2.13 Describe the principles of end-of-life care for patients, avoiding unnecessary investigations or treatment, and ensuring physical comforts by providing pain relief, psychosocial support and other elements of palliative care after discussion with their family carers.

2.14 Retrieve, interpret and record information effectively in clinical data systems.

3. Health and Society: the medical graduate as a health advocate

At the end of basic medical education, graduates are able to:

3.1 Accept responsibility to protect and advance the health and well-being of individuals, communities and populations.

3.2 Explain factors that contribute to health, illness, disease and success of treatment of populations, including issues relating to health inequities and inequalities, diversity of cultural, spiritual and community values, and socio-economic and physical environment factors.

3.3 Communicate effectively in wider roles including health advocacy.

3.4 Explain and evaluate common population health screening and prevention approaches, including the use of technology for surveillance and monitoring of the health status of populations, and provide instructions on patients' follow-up visits, medications and rehabilitative therapies, etc.

3.5 Understand the quality assurance system and safety management system of health care in hospitals, and be aware of their own competence, responsibilty and limits in medical practice. Attach importance to patients' safety, and recognize relevant risk factors in time.

3.6 Understand the structures and functions of the national health care system in China, and the roles and relationships between health agencies and services, and understand the principles of rational allocation of resources, to meet the needs of individuals, populations and national health systems.

3.7 Understand the global health issues and the determinants of health and diseases.

4. Professionalism: the medical graduate as a professional

At the end of basic medical education, graduates are able to:

4.1 Provide humanistic and quality health care services to all patients in accordance with the *Ethic Principles of Chinese Physicians*.

4.2 Demonstrate professional values in health practice, including empathy, respect for all patients and committement to high quality clinical service standards, and personal qualities of honest, integrity, teamwork and leadership.

4.3 Explain and apply the main principles of medical ethics in clinical practices. Communicate effectively with patients and their family members, colleagues and other health care professionals regarding ethical issues in medicine.

4.4 Be aware of the factors affecting physicians' health and well-being, such as fatigue, stress management and infection control, to mitigate health risks of professional practice, and identify the potential risks posed to patients by their own health.

4.5 Abide by the laws and regulations regarding clinical practiceas well as professional ethics.

4.6 Recognize the limits of their own expertise, and show respect for other health care professionals, to learn and work effectively as a team.

4.7 Demonstrate awareness of self-directed learning and lifelong learning. Recognize the importance of continuous self-improvement and demonstrate a commitment to excellence.

Standards for Basic Medical Education in China

1. Mission and Outcomes

1.1 Mission

Basic standards:

The medical school **must**

- state its mission and make it known to its stakeholders including the leadership, staff and students of the school and health sectors and etc. (B* 1.1.1)
- in its mission outline the objectives and the educational strategy in order to produce medical graduates meeting the graduate outcomes of basic medical education. (B 1.1.2)
- on the premise of abiding by relevant laws, in the mission encompass the health needs of the community, the needs of the health care system and

---

*: B refers to Basic Standards, similarly hereinafter

other aspects of social accountability. (B 1.1.3)

Quality development standards:

The medical school **should**

- ensure that the mission encompasses:
  - medical research attainment. (Q^* 1.1.1)
  - aspects of global health. (Q 1.1.2)

Annotations

- *Mission* illustrates the overarching framework of a medical school and its medical education program, including its positioning, educational philosophy and expected outcomes. It should match the resources and management of the school, while taking into consideration the local and national, regional and global expectations of medicine and the needs of development. It should also reflect the history, culture, and the development vision of the school. The positioning of the school should reflect its purpose, type and level of the education it provides, the community it serves and its development goals. The educational philosophy

---

*: Q refers to Quality Development Standards, similarly hereinafter

should reflect the concepts and ideas it upholds in the training of medical students.
- The *Medical school* is the educational organization providing basic education programs in medicine. The medical school can be an independent institution or part of or affiliated to a university. Medical schools would include university affiliated hospitals and other affiliated clinical facilities. Medical school not only provides basic medical education, medical research and medical services but also provides educational programs for other stages of medical education and for other health professions.
- *Health sectors* include the health care delivery system, whether public or private, and medical research institutions.
- *Encompassing the needs of health care system* refers to interaction with the local community, especially the health and health related sectors, and adjustment of the curriculum to demonstrate attention to and knowledge about health problems of the community.

- *Social accountability* refers to the willingness and ability to respond to the needs of society, of patients and the health and health related sectors and to contribute to the national and international development of medicine by fostering competencies in health care, medical education and medical research. This would be based on the school's own principles and in respect of the autonomy of universities. In matters outside its control especially health related issues, the medical school would still demonstrate social responsiveness by explaining relationships and drawing attention to consequences.
- *Medical research* would include all the scientific research related to medicine in the biomedical, clinical, behavioral and social sciences.
- *Aspects of global health* refers to the awareness of major international health priorities and concerns, including that of health consequences of inequality and injustice due to racial differences, regional and wealth disparity, and that of cross-disciplinary, cross-sector and cross-border health

management to address above challenges.

1.2 Participation in formulation of mission

Basic standards:

The medical school **must**

- ensure that its principal stakeholders on campus participate in formulating the mission. (B 1.2.1)

Quality development standards:

The medical school **should**

- ensure that the formulation of its mission is based also on input from other stakeholders. (Q 1.2.1)

Annotations

- *Principal stakeholders on campus* would include teachers, students, leadership and administrative staff of a university/school.
- *Other stakeholders* would include representatives of education and health care authorities, employers, the community and public (e.g. users of the health care delivery system, including patient organisations), academic and administrative staff, professional organisations, medical scientific bodies and postgraduate educators.

1.3 Institutional autonomy and academic freedom
Basic standards:
The medical school **must**
- have the autonomy to formulate and implement policies for which its faculty/academic staff and administration are responsible, especially regarding
  - design of the curriculum. (B 1.3.1)
  - allocation and use of the resources necessary for implementation of the curriculum. (B 1.3.2)
- obtain the academic support from the disciplines such as natural sciences, humanities and social sciences. (B 1.3.3)

Quality development standards:
The medical school **should**
- ensure academic freedom for its staff and students in regards to:
  - illustrating and analyzing issues of medicine from different perspectives in teaching and learning. (Q 1.3.1)
  - employing appropriate resources necessary for teaching and learning. (Q 1.3.2)

- exploring new research findings to illustrate specific problems. (Q 1.3.3)
- enhance the integration of humanities, social and natural sciences with the medical sciences. (Q 1.3.4)

Annotations

- *Institutional autonomy* would include appropriate independence from government and other counterparts (regional and local authorities, private co-operations, the professions, unions and other interest groups) to be able to make decisions in key areas such as student admission, design of curriculum, assessments, staff recruitment/ selection and employment conditions, research and resource allocation. Institutional autonomy should be respected on the premise of complying with laws and regulations and the developmental principles of medical education.
- *Academic freedom* would include appropriate freedom of expression, freedom of inquiry and publication for staff and students.

1.4 Educational outcomes
Basic standards:

The medical school **must**
- define the intended educational outcomes that students should exhibit upon graduation in relation to
  - requirements in the four domains of science and scholarship, clinical practice, health and society, and professionalism. (B 1.4.1)
  - appropriate foundation for future careers in any branch of medicine. (B 1.4.2)
  - their future roles in the health sector. (B 1.4.3)
  - their subsequent postgraduate training. (B 1.4.4)
  - their commitment to lifelong learning. (B 1.4.5)
  - the health needs of the community, the needs of the health care system and other aspects of social accountability. (B 1.4.6)
- ensure appropriate student conducts with respect to fellow students, faculty members, other health care professionals, patients and their families. (B 1.4.7)

Quality development standards:

The medical school **should**
- specify and co-ordinate the linkage of outcomes to be acquired by graduation with acquired outcomes in postgraduate training. (Q 1.4.1)
- specify requirements for and expected outcomes of student engagement in medical research. (Q 1.4.2)
- draw attention to global health related outcomes. (Q 1.4.3)

Annotations
- *Educational outcomes* refer to statements of science and scholarship, clinical practice, health and society, and professionalism that students demonstrate at the end of a period of learning, which include documented knowledge and understanding of (a) the basic biomedical sciences; (b) the preventive medicine including public health, health education and promotion; (c) the behavioral and social sciences, including medical ethics and health laws; (d) the clinical sciences, including clinical skills with respect

to diagnostic procedures, practical procedures, communication skills, therapies and prevention of diseases, health promotion, rehabilitation, clinical reasoning and problem solving; (e) the ability to undertake lifelong learning and demonstrate professionalism in connection with different roles of a physician, also in relation to the medical profession.

- *Appropriate student conducts* must be specified in the student manual and relevant documents.
- *Life-long learning* is the professional responsibility to keep up to date in knowledge and skills through assessments and reflection or recognized continuing professional development (CPD) or continuing medical education (CME) activities. CPD includes all activities that physicians undertake, formally and informally, to maintain, update, develop and enhance their knowledge, skills and attitudes in response to the needs of their patients. CPD is a broader concept than CME, which describes continuing education in the knowledge and skills of medical practice.

- *Global health* refers to the health-related issues with impacts across national boundaries and need to be addressed by international collaborations.

2. Education Programme

2.1 Curriculum design and instructional methods
Basic standards:
The medical school **must**
- make its curriculum suitable for the mission, objectives and educational outcomes of the school based upon the health needs of the community and society, reflecting the advances in medical sciences and the transforming trends of healthcare services. (B 2.1.1)
- ensure that the curriculum upholds the principles of strengthening foundational learning and skills training, emphasizing professionalism and personal quality development. (B 2.1.2)
- define the curricular models. (B 2.1.3)
- define the instructional and learning methods employed. (B 2.1.4)
- ensure that the curriculum prepares students

for lifelong learning and self-directed learning. (B 2.1.5)
- ensure that the curriculum is delivered in accordance with principles of equality. (B 2.1.6)

Quality development standards:

The medical school **should**

- use a curriculum and instructional/learning methods that stimulate, prepare and support students to take responsibility for their own learning process. (Q 2.1.1)

Annotations

- *Curriculum* in this document refers to the educational programme and it includes a statement of the intended educational outcomes, the contents/syllabi, experiences and processes of the programme, consisting of a description of the structure of the planned instructional and learning methods and assessment methods.
- *Curriculum models* would include models based on disciplines, organ systems, clinical problems/tasks or disease patterns.
- *Instructional and learning methods* encompass

lectures, small-group teaching, problem-based and case-based learning, peer assisted learning, laboratory exercises, clerkship and internship, bedside teaching, clinical demonstrations, clinical skills laboratory training, field exercises in the community and web-based instruction.
- *Principles of equality* mean equal treatment of staff and students irrespective of gender, ethnicity, religion, sexual orientation, socio-economic status, and taking into account physical capabilities.
- *The curriculum and instructional methods* would be based on contemporary learning principles.

2.2 Scientific method
Basic standards:
The medical school **must**
- throughout the curriculum teach
    - the principles of scientific methods, including analytical and critical thinking. (B 2.2.1)
    - medical research methods. (B 2.2.2)
    - evidence-based medicine. (B 2.2.3)

Quality development standards:

The medical school **should**

- encourage students to participate in research projects and include scientific research training throughout the curriculum. (Q 2.2.1)
- in the curriculum include elements of original or advanced research. (Q 2.2.2)
- integrate scientific and medical research method principles and the application of evidence-based medicine throughout the curriculum. (Q 2.2.3)

2.3 Behavioural and social sciences, medical ethics and natural sciences

Basic standards:

The medical school **must**

- in the curriculum identify and incorporate the contributions of:
  - behavioral sciences, social sciences, medical ethics and medical jurisprudence. (B 2.3.1)
  - natural sciences. (B 2.3.2)

Quality development standards:

The medical school **should**

- in the curriculum adjust and modify the contributions of the behavioral and social sciences as well as medical ethics to:

- scientific, technological and clinical developments. (Q 2.3.1)
- current and anticipated needs of the society and the health care system. (Q 2.3.2)
- changing demographic and cultural contexts. (Q 2.3.3)

Annotations

- *Behavioral and social sciences* would conform to the local needs, interests and traditions – include medical ethics, medical jurisprudence, medical psychology, medical sociology and health services administration. The content and depth of each course depend on programme objectives. The medical school is encouraged to integrate behavioral and social sciences effectively into the course contents of medical disciplines or other professional trainings.
- *Natural sciences* include mathematics, physics and chemistry, etc.

2.4 Basic biomedical sciences

Basic standards:

The medical school **must**

- in the curriculum identify and incorporate the contributions of the basic biomedical sciences to create understanding of scientific knowledge, concepts and methods fundamental to acquiring and applying clinical sciences. (B 2.4.1)

Quality development standards:

The medical school **should**

- in the curriculum adjust and modify the contributions of the biomedical sciences to the scientific, technological and clinical developments as well as current and anticipated needs of the society and the health care system. (Q 2.4.1)

Annotation

- *Basic biomedical sciences* would include core courses like human anatomy, histology and embryology, pathology, pathogenic biology, cell biology, medical genetics, biochemistry, physiology, medical immunology, pharmacology, pathophysiology and developing courses like molecular biology, neurobiology, biophysics and bioinformatics. All the above courses can also be presented in the form of integrated contents. Core courses are always the compulsory courses and developing courses can be compulsory or elective courses based on programme objectives.

2.5 Public health sciences

Basic standards:

The medical school **must**

- in the curriculum identify and incorporate the contributions of public health sciences to develop students' awareness of population health and disease prevention strategies, allowing them to function well in health education, promotion and management efforts. (B 2.5.1)

Quality development standards:

The medical school **should**

- ensure that the curriculum expands the students' vision in global health so the learners understand the global health issues and think in global health perspectives. (Q 2.5.1)

92   Standards for Basic Medical Education in China

Annotation

- *Public health sciences* include medical statistics, epidemiology, global health, health promotion and health education, maternal and child health care, child and adolescent health, social medicine, environmental health, nutrition and food hygiene, occupational health and occupational medicine.

2.6   Clinical sciences and skills

Basic standards:

The medical school **must**

- in the curriculum identify and incorporate the contributions of the clinical sciences to ensure that students spend the specified amount of time in training in major clinical disciplines and acquire sufficient knowledge and clinical and professional skills to assume appropriate responsibilities after graduation. (B 2.6.1)
- ensure that students spend a reasonable part of the programme in planned contact with patients in relevant clinical settings. (B 2.6.2)
- ensure the effective integration of medical knowledge and clinical clerkship. (B 2.6.3)

Standards for Basic Medical Education in China **93**

- ensure that each student completes his or her internship at a clinical site that has written agreement with the medical school and possesses appropriate teaching qualifications. (B 2.6.4)
- satisfy the time requirement of clinical internship prior to graduation, which is no less than 48 weeks, and cover major secondary disciplines such as internal medicine, surgery, pediatrics, gynecology and obstetrics in the internship. (B 2.6.5)
- organize clinical trainings with appropriate attention to patient and student safety. (B 2.6.6)
- in the curriculum identify and incorporate the contributions of communication skills related with the doctors' responsibilities to ensure that students communicate professionally with patients, their families, peers and other medical team members. (B 2.6.7)
- introduce the basic principles of traditional Chinese medicine in the curriculum. (B 2.6.8)
- encourage early exposure of students to patients in professional settings. (B 2.6.9)

94 Standards for Basic Medical Education in China

Quality development standards:

The medical school **should**

- ensure that each student has opportunities for early patient contact, and in a gradual manner, for participation in patient care under close supervision. (Q 2.6.1)

- structure different elements of clinical skills training according to the phases of student learning in the programme. (Q 2.6.2)

- provide students opportunities for interprofessional education (IPE) in which students learn teamwork from professionals of other medical specialties. (Q 2.6.3)

Annotations

- *The clinical sciences* would include core courses like diagnostics, internal medicine (neurological diseases and infectious diseases), surgery (general surgery and anesthesiology), gynecology, obstetrics, pediatrics, psychiatry, ophthalmology, otolaryngology and head and neck surgery, dermatovenerology, stomatology, traditional Chinese medicine or other ethno-medicine and general practice/family medicine;

and developing courses like emergency medicine, rehabilitation, geriatrics, oncology, palliative medicine, physical therapy, radiological treatment, clinical pharmacology (including the reasonable application of antibiotics). The courses for clinical medicine can also be presented as integrated course contents. Refer to 2.4 (basic biomedical sciences) for the meanings of core courses and developing courses.

- *Clinical skills* include history taking, physical examination, communication skills, auxiliary examination, clinical procedural performance, diagnosis and differentiated diagnosis, and prescription and treatment practices.
- *Professional skills* would include patient management skills, team-work/team leadership skills, and inter-professional trainings.
- *A reasonable part* would mean the fact that the clinical teaching time is no less than half of the programme and that the contact with patients in the clinical settings accounts for no less than one third of the programme.

96 Standards for Basic Medical Education in China

- *Clinical sites with teaching qualification* indicate qualified teaching hospitals that have been accredited by education and/or health authorities.

- *Major secondary disciplines* in the internship would include internal medicine (with respiratory, cardiovascular and gastrointestinal medicine for no less than 3 weeks respectively), surgery (with general surgery including gastrointestinal and hepatobiliary for no less than 6 weeks), gynecology and obstetrics, and pediatrics.

- *Patient and student safety* would require close supervision of clinical activities conducted by students and provide safe learning environment for students.

- *Early patient contact* would partly take place in primary care settings and would primarily include history taking, physical examination and communication with patients, families and healthcare professionals.

2.7 Curriculum structure, composition and duration

Basic standards:

The medical school **must**

Standards for Basic Medical Education in China   **97**

- describe the content, extent and sequencing of courses and other curricular elements to ensure appropriate coordination between basic biomedical, behavioral and social, and clinical subjects. (B 2.7.1)
- allow optional (elective) courses and define the balance between the core and optional courses as part of the educational programme. (B 2.7.2)

Quality development standards:

The medical school **should**

- in the curriculum:
  - ensure horizontal integration of associated sciences, disciplines and subjects. (Q 2.7.1)
  - ensure vertical integration of the clinical sciences with the basic biomedical and the behavioural and social sciences. (Q 2.7.2)
  - introduce complementary medicine and their roles. (Q 2.7.3)

Annotations

- Examples of *horizontal integration* would be integrating basic biomedical sciences such as anatomy, biochemistry and physiology or integrating disciplines of medicine and surgery such as medical and surgical gastroenterology or nephrology and urology.

- Examples of *vertical integration* would be integrating metabolic disorders with biochemistry or cardiology as in cardiovascular physiology.
- *Complementary medicine* would include traditional or alternative therapeutic practices. In general, it includes traditional Chinese medicine, Mongolian medicine and Tibetan medicine, as well as non-traditional medicine like health food and food therapies.

2.8 Programme management

Basic standards:

The medical school **must**

- have a curriculum committee, which under the governance of the academic leadership (the Dean) has the responsibility and authority for planning and implementing the curriculum to secure its intended educational outcomes. (B 2.8.1)
- in its curriculum committee ensure proper representation of staff and students. (B 2.8.2)

Quality development standards:

The medical school **should**

- through its curriculum committee plan and implement innovations in the curriculum. (Q 2.8.1)
- in its curriculum committee include representatives of other stakeholders. (Q 2.8.2)

Annotations

- *The authority of the curriculum committee* would include authority over specific departmental and disciplinary interests, and the control of the curriculum within existing rules and regulations as defined by the governance structure of the institutions and governmental authorities. The curriculum committee would allocate the granted resources for planning and implementing methods of teaching and learning, assessment of students and course evaluations.
- *Other stakeholders* would include other participants in the educational process, representing the teaching hospitals, clinical facilities, alumni, other health professions or faculties in the university. Other stakeholders might also include groups

representing the community and public (e.g. users of the healthcare delivery system, including patient organizations).

2.9 Linkage with medical practice and the health sector

Basic standards:

The medical school **must**

- ensure operational linkage between the educational programme and the subsequent stages of training or practice after graduation, making it possible for the graduates to receive continuous medical education. (B 2.9.1)

Quality development standards:

The medical school **should**

- ensure that the curriculum committee seeks input from institutions in which graduates will be expected to work, and modify the programme accordingly, and considers programme modification in response to feedback from the community and society. (Q 2.9.1)

Annotation

- *The operational linkage* implies identifying healthcare needs and defining required educational outcomes. This requires clear definition and description of the elements within the educational programmes and their inter-relationships in the various stages of training and practice, paying attention to the local, national, regional and global context. It would include mutual feedback to and from the health sector and participation of teachers and students in activities of the health team. Operational linkage also implies constructive dialogue with potential employers of the graduates as the basis for career guidance.

3. Assessment of Students

3.1 Assessment methods

Basic standards:

The medical school **must**

- define, state and publish the principles, methods and practices used for assessment of its students, including the type and frequency of assessment the criteria for setting pass marks, composition of marks, grade boundaries and number of allowed retakes. (B 3.1.1)

102 Standards for Basic Medical Education in China

- ensure that assessment covers the areas of science and scholarship, clinical practice, health and society, professionalism. (B 3.1.2)
- use a wide range of assessment methods and formats depending on different objectives. (B 3.1.3)
- use a system for appeal of assessment results. (B 3.1.4)

Quality development standards:

The medical school **should**

- actively initiate research of its assessment system and methods, and incorporate new assessment methods where appropriate. (Q 3.1.1)
- ensure that assessments are open to scrutiny by external experts. (Q 3.1.2)

3.2   Relationship between assessment and learning

Basic standards:

The medical school **must**

- use assessment principles, methods and practices that
    - ensure that the intended educational outcomes are met by the students. (B 3.2.1)
    - promote student learning. (B 3.2.2)

Standards for Basic Medical Education in China **103**

- provide an appropriate balance of formative and summative assessments to guide both learning and decisions about academic progress. (B 3.2.3)

Quality development standards:

The medical school **should**

- adjust the number and nature of examination of curricular elements to encourage both acquisition of the knowledge base and integrated learning. (Q 3.2.1)
- ensure timely, specific, constructive and fair feedback to students on the basis of assessment results. (Q 3.2.2)

Annotations

- *Assessment principles, methods and practices* would include consideration of number, time of examinations and other tests, balance between written and oral examinations, use of normative and criterion referenced judgements, and use of special types of examinations, e.g. objective structured clinical examination (OSCE), or mini clinical evaluation exercise (Mini-CEX), direct observation of procedural skills (DOPS) and computer-based case simulations (CCS).

- *Summative assessment* is performed after the educational activities, which is used to determine whether the education objectives have been achieved. Summative assessment focuses on the evaluation of performances and learning outcomes.

- *Formative assessment* stresses the combination of education and evaluation procedures, attaches importance to and emphasizes the timely feedback and modification during the course of teaching and learning. Formative assessment is both helpful for the teachers to know their teaching effectiveness and optimize teaching, and for the students to evaluate their own progress in learning and adjust their learning strategies accordingly.

- *Integrated learning* would include consideration of using integrated assessment, while ensuring reasonable tests of knowledge of individual disciplines or subject areas.

3.3 Analysis and feedback of assessment results

Basic standards:

The medical school **must**

- analyze the assessment results based on the educational measurement after all the examinations are finished. (B 3.3.1)
- provide feedback to students, faculty and academic affairs administrators. (B 3.3.2)

Quality development standards:

The medical school **should**

- apply the analyzed results in the improvement of teaching and learning. (Q 3.3.1)
- enhance the reform efforts and research of assessments. (Q 3.3.2)

Annotation

- *Analysis of assessment results* includes the degree of difficulties, differentiation, reliability, validity, content coverage, and student performance scores of the tests.

4. Students

4.1 Admission policy and selection

Basic standards:

The medical school **must**

- formulate an admission plan based on the national admission policy and periodically review it for adjustment. (B 4.1.1)
- pay attention to the diversity of students on the premise of guaranteeing the quality of enrolled students. (B 4.1.2)
- have no discrimination and bias under the condition of meeting the requirements of the program. (B 4.1.3)
- make the admission policies known to the public, including the school prospectus, programs, admission plan, tuition and fees, scholarships, and mechanism for appeal, etc., and describe the process of student selection and make the curriculum known to the applicants on the internet. (B 4.1.4)
- have a policy and implement a practice for transfer of students from other programmes and institutions. (B 4.1.5)

Standards for Basic Medical Education in China   **107**

Quality development standards:

The medical school **should**

- state clearly the relationship between student selection and the mission of the school, the educational programme and desired qualities of graduates. (Q 4.1.1)

- use a system for appeal of admission decisions. (Q 4.1.2)

Annotations

- *Admission plan* would imply adherence to the national regulations and policies to ensure the fair and equal treatments of students in the educational process.

- *The process of selection* would include both rationale and methods of student admissions such as the use of high school performance scores, other relevant academic or educational experiences, college entrance examination scores and student performance in interviews, including the evaluation of student motivations to become doctors, participation in social service projects and psychological tests. Selection would also take into account the differences in admission standards due to ethnic diversities and variations related to distinctive medical practices.

4.2 Student intake

Basic standards:

The medical school **must**

- define the size of student intake based on relevant national policies, the health needs of the community and society, and the educational resources of the school. (B 4.2.1)

Quality development standards:

The medical school **should**

- take the advice of stakeholders into consideration when reviewing and adjusting the size of student intake. (Q 4.2.1)

Annotations

- *The health needs of the community and society* would include consideration of national and regional demands for medical workforce as well as gender, ethnicity and other social requirements (socio-cultural and linguistic characteristics of the population), including the potential need of a special recruitment, admission and induction policy for underprivileged students and minorities.

- *Educational resources* would include the consideration of shared use of clinical education resources by the students of other health related programs.
- *Stakeholders* would include the education and health authorities, health facilities, faculty and students, and representatives of the public.

4.3 Student counseling and support

Basic standards:

The medical school **must**

- have a system for academic counseling and support of its student population. (B 4.3.1)
- offer support and guidance to students in their activities of learning, living, taking part-time jobs and choosing careers. (B 4.3.2)
- have an effective system of psychological counseling. (B 4.3.3)
- allocate resources for student support. (B 4.3.4)
- ensure confidentiality in relation to counseling and support. (B 4.3.5)

110   Standards for Basic Medical Education in China

Quality development standards:

The medical school **should**

- offer individualized academic guidance and counseling based on the student progress in learning. (Q 4.3.1)
- offer students career guidance and planning. (Q 4.3.2)

Annotations

- *Academic counseling* would include questions related to choice of electives, residency preparation and career guidance, etc.
- *Student support* would include medical services, career guidance, suitable accommodation for students with disabilities, and implementation of a student aid system offering scholarships, loans, subsidies and allowances for disadvantaged students in need of financial assistance.
- *Individualized academic guidance and counseling* would include appointing academic mentors for individual students or small groups of students.

4.4　Student representation

Basic standards:

The medical school **must**

- formulate and implement a policy, that ensures the participation of student representatives and appropriate participation in the design, management and evaluation of the curriculum, and in other matters relevant to students. (B 4.4.1)

- support students to establish student organizations allowed by law, guide and encourage organized student activities in providing equipment, spaces, and technical and financial support. (B 4.4.2)

Quality development standards:

The medical school **should**

- have student representatives serving in relevant committees, bodies of the school and organizations of the community and ensure that they have certain roles to play. (Q 4.4.1)

Annotation

- *Student organizations* would include relevant bodies for student self governance, self education and self service.

5. Academic Staff/Faculty

5.1 Recruitment and selection policy

Basic standards:

The medical school **must**

- formulate and implement a staff qualification certification and selection system, to make sure that the teachers meet the performance demands in teaching, research and service functions. (B 5.1.1)

- have a well-structured faculty team composed of a sufficient number of qualified academic staff/faculty based on the school mission and scale. (B 5.1.2)

- outline the responsibilities of the academic staff/ faculty to ensure an appropriate ratio and balance between teaching, research and service functions. (B 5.1.3)

- set merit criteria for teaching, research and services, and evaluate the performance of the academic staff/faculty regularly. (B 5.1.4)

- have a corresponding mechanism to ensure that the results of teacher performance evaluation play a role in school decisions for promotions and appointments of academic, administrative or entitlement nature. (B 5.1.5)

Quality development standards:

The medical school **should**

- in its policy for staff recruitment and selection take into account the school mission and the requirements for reform and development. (Q 5.1.1)
- take into account the reasonable and effective utilization of personnel, funds and resources when formulating the selection policy to ensure the balanced development of teaching, research and service functions. (Q 5.1.2)

Annotations

- *Recruitment and selection policy* would include consideration of ensuring a sufficient number of highly qualified basic biomedical scientists, behavioural and social scientists and clinicians to deliver the curriculum.
- *Qualified academic staff/faculty* would indicate that the academic staff/faculty should possess good professional ethics and the scholarship and teaching ability that match their academic

ranks, deliver corresponding courses and assume required teaching assignments, and be certified by the corresponding educational authorities. Non-medical staff should have the necessary knowledge of medical education.

- *Merits* would be measured by formal qualifications, professional experience, teaching awards, research output, student evaluation and peer recognition.

5.2 Staff activity and staff development

Basic standards:

The medical school **must**

- formulate and effectively implement policies related to faculty training, development, support and appraisal, to ensure that the central focus is on educating students. These policies should
  - guarantee the legal rights of the academic staff/ faculty. (B 5.2.1)
  - recognize and support the professional development of the academic staff/faculty. (B 5.2.2)
  - encourage that the academic staff/faculty apply their clinical experience and research findings in teaching. (B 5.2.3)

Standards for Basic Medical Education in China **115**

- ensure that the academic staff/faculty can be directly involved in the curriculum design and the decision-making process related to educational management. (B 5.2.4)
- ensure sufficient knowledge by individual staff members of education objectives and the curriculum. (B 5.2.5)
- make efforts to promote the communication among the academic staff/faculty. (B 5.2.6)
- ensure that the academic staff/faculty possess and maintain their competence in teaching. (B 5.2.7)
- allow a balance of faculty roles in teaching, research and service functions. (B 5.2.8)

Quality development standards:

The medical school **should**

- attach importance to the differences in courses and teaching models and reasonably allocate the academic staff/faculty based on the requirements of the curriculum. (Q 5.2.1)
- establish a mechanism for the academic staff/ faculty to participate in the management and

policy-making of the school/university. (Q 5.2.2)

Annotations

- *Staff activity and development* would involve not only new teachers, but also all the teachers in basic biomedical sciences and the clinical sciences.

- *Staff development* would emphasize the promotion of teaching abilities. The departments for teacher support and development can provide training in educational theory, curriculum design, teaching methods and teacher evaluations.

- *Decision-making process related to educational management* would include having roles to shape decisions on student admission and services. The school should also ensure that teachers also take part in the decision-making of other important issues.

- *Sufficient knowledge by individual staff members of the curriculum* would include knowledge about instructional pedagogies, overall curricular contents, and assessment methods, for the purpose of fostering the cooperation of teachers and teaching content integration among different disciplines, and offering students appropriate guidance for learning.

- *Communication among the academic staff/ faculty* would include interdisciplinary and cross-disciplinary communications, and in particular, the communications between teachers of the basic medical sciences and the clinical sciences.

- *Competence in teaching* would include adapting to the educational objectives of the school, following its basic principles, designing appropriate teaching activities, and choosing student assessment methods.

- *A balance of faculty roles in teaching, research and service functions* would include provision of protected time for each function. *Service functions* would include clinical duties in the health care delivery system, student guidance, participation in governance and management and other social services as well.

6. Educational Resources

6.1 Education budgets and allocation of resources

Basic standards:

The medical school **must**

- have sufficient financial support and reliable access to fund raising. (B 6.1.1)
- have the financial resources to sustain a sound program of medical education and institutional goals. (B 6.1.2)

Quality development standards:

The medical school **should**

- derive the present and anticipated financial resources from diverse sources. (Q 6.1.1)
- support research and implementation of medical education reforms financially. (Q 6.1.2)

Annotations

- In the *financial resources*, the tuition charged by the medical school must be managed and used according to national regulations. The funds used for teaching and their proportion in the annual final account of the school must meet national regulations. The expenditures of educational funds should have an annual increase to ensure steady educational development.

- *Derive the present and anticipated financial resources from diverse sources* would include government appropriation, tuitions, investments made by civic organizations and private citizens, donations and funds, supports of affiliated and teaching hospitals, incomes from school-run enterprises and social services, etc.

6.2 Physical facilities

Basic standards:

The medical school **must**

- have sufficient physical facilities for staff and students to ensure that the curriculum can be delivered effectively. (B 6.2.1)
- ensure a learning environment, which is safe for staff, students and patients. (B 6.2.2)
- provide sites and equipment for simulated clinical training to students. (B 6.2.3)

120   Standards for Basic Medical Education in China

Quality development standards:

The medical school **should**

- improve the learning environment by regularly updating and modifying or extending the physical facilities to match the developments of education programs. (Q 6.2.1)

- update and effectively utilize simulated clinical training equipment to develop simulation-based clinical pedagogies. (Q 6.2.2)

Annotations

- *Physical facilities* would include all types of class-rooms, multimedia equipment, tutorial rooms, laboratories, equipment, specimen and consumable material for basic medical sciences, clinical skills center and simulation equipment, clinical demonstration rooms, libraries, information technology and network resources. School should also provide student amenities including accommodation and recreational facilities for students.

- *A safe learning environment* would include provisions of necessary information and protection from harmful substances, specimens and organisms, laboratory safety regulations and safety equipment. A medical school publishes policies and procedures to ensure student safety and to address emergency and disaster preparedness.

6.3 Clinical training resources

Basic standards:

The medical school **must**

- have tertiary class-A affiliated hospitals as clinical teaching sites. (B 6.3.1)
- have sufficient clinical teaching sites to ensure adequate clinical experience and necessary resources in clinical teaching, including sufficient patients and clinical training facilities. The number of students in the medical specialties and the number of patient beds in these hospitals should have a ratio of less than 1:1. (B 6.3.2)
- have enough staff from appropriate disciplines, and with the necessary skills and experience to deliver teaching and support students' learning. (B 6.3.3)

122 Standards for Basic Medical Education in China

Quality development standards:

The medical school **should**

- continuously evaluate, adapt and improve clinical training resources to meet the needs of teaching and healthcare services. (Q 6.3.1)

Annotations

- *Affiliated hospitals* are subsidaries of the medical school, which are under the direct control of the medical school.

- *Clinical teaching sites* encompass teaching hospitals, training hospitals and community health centers in addition to the affiliated hospitals. A teaching hospital must meet the following requirements: governmental documents certifying it as a clinical teaching site of a medical school; written agreements between the medical school and the hospital; be capable of and responsible for delivering the medical courses such as lectures, tutorials and internship. A clinical teaching site must have specialized organizations and staff in charge of the administration and management of clinical trainings.

Standards for Basic Medical Education in China **123**

- *Clinical teaching resources* also include adequate numbers of patients with wide range of diseases, in addtion to pedagogical equipment.
- *Medical specialties* in this document refer to the medical specialties that award the degree of Bachelor of Medicine, including clinical medicine, stomatology, anesthesiology, medical radiology, ophthalmology and optometry, psychiatry, radioactive medicine, traditional Chinese medicine, clinical discipline of Chinese and western integrative medicine, basic medicine, forensic medicine and preventive medicine. The students of medical specialties include undergraduate students from the above specialties, overseas students taught in Chinese/ English and junior college students.
- *Patient beds* refer to the total in affiliated hospitals and teaching hospitals. The patient beds in affiliated hospital refer to the sum of them in the affiliated comprehensive hospitals and specialized hospitals responsible for clinical teaching and practices. The patient beds in teaching hospitals

refer to the number of beds in the teaching hospitals responsible for the whole process of clinical teaching, clerkship and internship and the hospitals should also possess graduate students of clinical medicine, but the patient beds in the specialized hospitals are excluded. The number of patient beds is recognized as the number in the official reports of the hospital submitted to the health authorities at the end of the previous year. The number of patient beds should be the smaller one of the number registered and the number used.

• *Evaluation of clinical training resources* would include the assessment in regards of settings, equipment, number and categories of patients, as well as health practices, supervision and administration to measure whether they meet the teaching requirements. The resources in the affiliated and teaching hospitals shared by students from other medical schools should also be considered.

6.4 Information technology

Basic standards:

The medical school **must**

- own adequate information and communication technology infrastructure and support systems. (B 6.4.1)
- formulate and implement policies which address the effective use of information and communication technology and resources in medical education to ensure the delivery of the educational program. (B 6.4.2)

Quality development standards:

The medical school **should**

- enable teachers and students to use existing and explore appropriate new information technology to support self-directed learning. (Q 6.4.1)
- optimise student access to relevant patient data and health care information systems. (Q 6.4.2)

Annotation

- *Effective use of information and communication technology* would include the use of computers, internal and external networks and other means.

126 Standards for Basic Medical Education in China

This would include coordination with library resources and IT services of the institution. The policy would include common access to all educational items through a learning management system. Information and communication technology would be useful for preparing students for evidence-based medicine and life-long learning through continuing professional development (CPD)/ continuing medical education (CME).

6.5 Educational expertise

Basic standards:

The medical school **must**

- formulate and implement a policy that have access to educational expertise involved in deciding on important issues concerning medical education, including developing and adjusting the educational curriculum and teaching and assessment methods. (B 6.5.1)

Quality development standards:

The medical school **should**

- allow the educational experts to play an important role in faculty development. (Q 6.5.1)

- pay attention to the development of in-house expertise in program evaluations and in research on medical education . (Q 6.5.2)

Annotation

- *Educational expertise* would rely on experts who had experience studying and solving problems in medical education and these experts would include teachers, medical doctors, administrators and researchers with research experience in medical education. It can be provided by an education development unit or a team of interested and experienced teachers at the institution or be acquired from another national or international institution.

6.6 Educational exchanges

Basic standards:

The medical school **must**

- formulate and implement a policy for national and international collaboration with other educational institutions. (B 6.6.1)
- facilitate regional and international exchange of staff and students by providing appropriate resources. (B 6.6.2)

128 Standards for Basic Medical Education in China

Quality development standards:

The medical school **should**

- formulate and implement a policy for transfer of educational credits. (Q 6.6.1)
- ensure that exchange is purposefully organized, taking into account the needs of staff and students, respecting the customs of each teaching site and following ethical principles. (Q 6.6.2)

Annotation

- *A policy for transfer of educational credits* would be facilitated by establishing agreements on mutual recognition of educational elements and through active programme coordination between medical schools. It would also be facilitated with the use of a transparent system of credit units and flexible interpretation of course requirements.

7. Programme Evaluation

7.1 Mechanisms for programme monitoring and evaluation

Basic standards:

The medical school **must**

- establish a mechanism for programme monitoring and evaluation with emphasis on the monitoring and evaluation of curricula, educational process and outcome. (B 7.1.1)
- establish detailed requirements for all educational components according to the quality standards of medical specialties. (B 7.1.2)
- ensure the relevant results of evaluation influence the curriculum. (B 7.1.3)
- enable the faculty, students and administrators to understand the system of education program monitoring and evaluation. (B 7.1.4)

Quality development standards:

The medical school **should**

- periodically evaluate the programme by comprehensively addressing the context of the educational process, the specific components of the curriculum, the long-term outcomes acquired, and its social accountability. (Q 7.1.1)
- follow up student progress, such as learning processes, changes in learning abilities, and student life and academic assistance, and give

130 Standards for Basic Medical Education in China

timely feedback to the students. (Q 7.1.2)

- arrange training for related personnel in charge of the evaluation, so that they are able to choose and use appropriate and effective evaluation methods. (Q 7.1.3)

Annotations

- *Programme evaluation* is the process of systematic gathering of information to judge the effectiveness and adequacy of educational programme, educational process and long-term outcomes, so as to provide references for the improvement of education quality and making decisions on education issues. It would imply the use of reliable and valid methods of data collection and analysis. The information and data may include the quality evaluation documents of universities or medical school, such as rules and policies, brochures, meeting minutes, joint agreements with other educational institutions, supervisory reports and student evaluation results, etc.

- *Programme monitoring* would imply the routine

collection of data about key aspects of the curriculum for the purpose of ensuring that the educational process is on track and for identifying any areas in need of intervention.

- *The context of the educational process* would include the organization and resources as well as the learning environment and culture of the medical school.

- *Specific components of the curriculum* would include course description, teaching and learning pedagogies, clinical rotations and assessment methods.

- *Long-term outcomes acquired* would be measured by e.g. results at national licensing examinations, qualifying examinations for standardized training of residents, career choices, employer comments on performance of graduates, etc, and these would provide the basis for curricular improvement.

7.2 Teacher and student feedback

Basic standards:

The medical school **must**

- apply multiple evaluation methods, systematically

seek and analyse information, and give feedback to teachers and students. (B 7.2.1)

Quality development standards:

The medical school **should**

- use feedback results for programme development and achieve expected improvement. (Q 7.2.1)

Annotation

- *Feedback* would include information about the processes and outcomes of the educational programmes. It would also include information about school policies and regulations malpractices or inappropriate conducts involving teachers or students with or without legal consequences.

7.3 Performance of students and graduates

Basic standards:

The medical school **must**

- analyse performance of cohorts of students and graduates in relation to its mission, intended educational outcomes, curriculum, and provision of resources. (B 7.3.1)

Quality development standards:

The medical school **should**

- use the results of student performance evaluations to shape admission policies, revise education programs and offer consultation services to students. (Q 7.3.1)

Annotation

- Measures of *performance of graduate cohorts* would include information about career choice, performance in clinical service delivery and post-graduation promotion as well as other job performance measures for graduates.

7.4 Involvement of stakeholders

Basic standards:

The medical school **must**

- in its programme monitoring and evaluation activities involve its principal stakeholders on campus such as academic staff, students and administrators. (B7.4.1)

Quality development standards:

The medical school **should**

- encourage other stakeholders to contribute to its

course and programme evaluation and have access to the evaluation results. (Q 7.4.1)

- seek other stakeholders' feedback on the performance of graduates and on the curriculum. (Q 7.4.2)

Annotation

- *Other stakeholders* would include other representatives of academic and administrative staff, representatives of the community and public (e.g. users of the health care system), education and health care authorities, professional organizations, medical scientific bodies and postgraduate educators.

8. Scientific Research

8.1 Education and scientific research
Basic standards:
The medical school **must**

- formulate and implement a policy that promotes the coordinated development of scientific research and education programs. (B 8.1.1)
- use scientific research and scholarship as a basis for curricular development and implementation.

(B 8.1.2)

- strengthen the study of medical education and management, to provide theoretical basis for the educational reform and development. (B 8.1.3)

Quality development standards:

The medical school **should**

- incorporate scientific research activities and outcomes into the educational process, to train students' ability in scientific thinking, scientific methods and spirits of science, and to ensure positive interactions of scientific research and education activities. (Q 8.1.1)

Annotation

- *Scientific research* encompasses the scientific activities in biomedical, clinical, behavioral and social sciences. Its influence on current teaching would facilitate teaching of scientific methods and evidence-based medicine.

8.2   Scientific research by staff

Basic standards:

The medical school **must**

- encourage academic staff to conduct scientific

research and provide basic resources needed for the complementary development of scientific research and education. (B 8.2.1)

- ensure academic staff to be equipped with corresponding ability in scientific research. (B 8.2.2)

Quality development standards:

The medical school **should**

- encourage the active involvement of academic staff in the research of medical education, so as to enhance the teaching effectiveness. (Q 8.2.1)

8.3   Scientific research of students

Basic standards:

The medical school **must**

- use the scientific research activities as an important pathway to cultivate students' scientific literacy and creativity, and adopt effective measures to provide students with opportunities and resources needed for scientific research. (B 8.3.1)
- actively engage in activities which are instrumental in cultivating students' research competencies, such as incorporating comprehensive experiments and self-designed experiments in the curriculum, holding

academic lectures and organizing scientific research teams. (B 8.3.2)

Quality development standards:

The medical school **should**

- provide funds for the scientific research activities of students. (Q 8.3.1)

9. Governance and Administration

9.1 Governance

Basic standards:

The medical school **must**

- define its governance structures and functions including their relationships within the university, and establish an effective management mechanism among university, medical school and affiliated hospitals, so as to ensure the coordinated development of healthcare delivery, education and research. (B 9.1.1)

- establish functional committees in its governance structures to review and discuss important issues involving the curriculum, educational reform and scientific research. The committees should include principal stakeholders on campus such as the school leaders, representatives of teachers and students, and administrative staff. (B 9.1.2)

Quality development standards:

The medical school **should**

- in its corresponding committees include other stakeholders such as relevant governmental authorities and regulatory bodies, education and health care sectors, and representatives of the community and public. (Q 9.1.1)
- ensure transparency of the work of governance and its decisions. (Q 9.1.2)

Annotations

- *Governance* is primarily concerned with policy making, the processes of establishing general institutional and programme policies and also with control of the implementation of the policies. The institutional and programme policies would normally encompass decisions on the mission of the medical school, the curriculum, admission policy, staff recruitment and selection policy and decisions on interaction and linkage with medical practice and the health sector as well as other external relations.

- *Members of the committees* should be widely representative. The activities of the committees should be organized by the persons in charge, and recorded in details concerning the time, issues discussed, decisions and participants.

- *Transparency* would be obtained by newsletters, web-information or disclosure of meeting minutes.

9.2   Academic leadership

Basic standards:

The medical school **must**

- clearly illustrate the management responsibilities and authority of its academic leadership on medical education, and ensure the execution accordingly. (B 9.2.1)

- ensure that the leadership responsible for education is relatively stable. (B 9.2.2)

- pay attention to the professional education background of the leaders in charge of medical education. (B 9.2.3)

140 Standards for Basic Medical Education in China

Quality development standards:

The medical school **should**

- periodically evaluate its academic leadership in relation to achievement of its mission and intended educational outcomes. (Q 9.2.1)

Annotations

- *Academic leadership* refers to the positions and persons within the governance and management structures being responsible for decisions on academic matters in teaching, research and service, and would include dean, vice deans, provost, etc.

- *Management responsibilities and authority* emphasize especially on the rights of leaders in charge of teaching affairs involving formulating and implementing the curriculum, and rationally allocating education resources.

9.3　Administrative staff and management

Basic standards:

The medical school **must**

- have an administrative staff with effective management structures and advanced educational philosophy that is appropriate to support implementation of its curricular and related activities. (B 9.3.1)

- establish a sound management system and operating procedures to ensure rational deployment of resources. (B 9.3.2)

Quality development standards:

The medical school **should**

- formulate and implement an internal programme of quality assurance on the management including regular reviews. (Q 9.3.1)

Annotations

- *Internal programme of quality assurance* would include consideration of the needs for improvements and review of the management.

9.4 Interaction with health sector

Basic standards:

The medical school **must**

- have constructive interaction and communication with the health related sectors for support to medical education. (B 9.4.1)

- sign agreements with relevant health sectors, so as

142 Standards for Basic Medical Education in China

to ensure the successful delivery of the curricula. (B 9.4.2)

Quality development standards:

The medical school **should**

- formalise extensive cooperation and exchanges with medical and health related sectors, so as to ensure a sustainable development. (Q 9.4.1)

Annotations

- *Relevant health sectors* would include the healthcare delivery system, whether public or private, medical research institutions, institutions and regulatory bodies with implications for health promotion and disease prevention.
- To *formalise extensive cooperation and exchanges* would mean entering into formal agreements, stating the content and forms of collaboration, and/or establishing joint projects.

10. Continuous Development

Basic standards:

The medical school **must**

- regularly review and evaluate self-development,

understand its own problems and make continuous improvement. (B 10.0.1)

Quality development standards:

The medical school **should**

- base the process of continuous development on prospective studies and analyses and on results of local evaluation and the literature on medical education. (Q 10.0.1)

- ensure that the process of continuous development and restructuring leads to the revision of its policies and practices in accordance with past experience, present activities and future perspectives. (Q 10.0.2)

- address the following issues in its process of development:

  - adaptation of mission statement and outcomes to the scientific, socio-economic and cultural development of the society. (Q 10.0.3)

  - modification of the intended educational outcomes of the graduating students in accordance with documented needs of the environment they will enter. The modification might include clinical skills, public health training and involvement in patient care appropriate to responsibilities encountered upon graduation. (Q 10.0.4)

- adaptation of the curriculum model and instructional methods to ensure that these are appropriate and relevant. (Q 10.0.5)

- adjustment of curricular elements and their relationships in keeping with developments in the basic biomedical, clinical, behavioral and social sciences, changes in the demographic profile and health/disease pattern of the population, and socioeconomic and cultural conditions. The adjustment would ensure that new relevant knowledge, concepts and methods are included and outdated ones are discarded. (Q 10.0.6)

- development of assessment principles, and methods and the number of examinations based on changes in intended educational outcomes and instructional methods. (Q 10.0.7)

- adaptation of student recruitment policy, selection methods and enrollment to changing expectations and circumstances, human resource needs, and requirements of the educational programme. (Q 10.0.8)

- adaptation of academic staff recruitment and development policy, updating of educational resources and optimizing the organizational structure and management according to changing needs. (Q 10.0.9)

- refinement of the process of programme monitoring and evaluation, so that the evaluation results are able to demonstrate the achievement of teaching objectives in time. (Q 10.0.10)